OXFORD MEDICAL PUBLICATIONS

Hypertension

Oxford Specialist Handbooks published and forthcoming

General Oxford Specialist Handbooks
A Resuscitation Room Guide
Addiction Medicine
Perioperative Medicine, Second Edition
Post-Operative Complications, Second Edition
Pulmonary Hypertension
Renal Transplantation

Oxford Specialist Handbooks in Anaesthesia
Cardiac Anaesthesia
Day Case Surgery
General Thoracic Anaesthesia
Neuroanaethesia
Obstetric Anaesthesia
Paediatric Anaesthesia
Regional Anaesthesia, Stimulation and Ultrasound Techniques

Oxford Specialist Handbooks in Cardiology
Adult Congenital Heart Disease
Cardiac Catheterization and Coronary Intervention
Cardiac Electrophysiology
Cardiovascular Magnetic Resonance
Echocardiography
Fetal Cardiology
Heart Failure
Nuclear Cardiology
Pacemakers and ICDs
Valvular Heart Disease

Oxford Specialist Handbooks in Critical Care
Advanced Respiratory Critical Care

Oxford Specialist Handbooks in End of Life Care
End of Life Care in Dementia
End of Life Care in Nephrology
End of Life in the Intensive Care Unit

Oxford Specialist Handbooks in Neurology
Epilepsy
Parkinson's Disease and Other Movement Disorders
Stroke Medicine

Oxford Specialist Handbooks in Paediatrics
Paediatric Dermatology
Paediatric Endocrinology and Diabetes
Paediatric Gastroenterology, Hepatology, and Nutrition
Paediatric Haematology and Oncology
Paediatric Intensive Care
Paediatric Nephrology
Paediatric Neurology
Paediatric Palliative Care
Paediatric Radiology
Paediatric Respiratory Medicine

Oxford Specialist Handbooks in Psychiatry
Child and Adolescent Psychiatry
Old Age Psychiatry

Oxford Specialist Handbooks in Radiology
Interventional Radiology
Musculoskeletal Imaging
Pulmonary Imaging

Oxford Specialist Handbooks in Surgery
Cardiothoracic Surgery
Colorectal Surgery
Hand Surgery
Liver and Pancreatobiliary Surgery
Operative Surgery, Second Edition
Oral Maxillofacial Surgery
Otolaryngology and Head and Neck Surgery
Paediatric Surgery
Plastic and Reconstructive Surgery
Surgical Oncology
Urological Surgery
Vascular Surgery

Oxford Specialist Handbooks

Hypertension

Joseph Cheriyan

Consultant Physician and Clinical Pharmacologist,
Clinical Pharmacology Unit,
University of Cambridge,
Cambridge, UK

Carmel M. McEniery

Senior Research Associate,
Clinical Pharmacology Unit,
University of Cambridge,
Cambridge, UK

Ian B. Wilkinson

Senior Lecturer,
Honorary Consultant Physician and
Clinical Pharmacologist,
Clinical Pharmacology Unit,
University of Cambridge,
Cambridge, UK

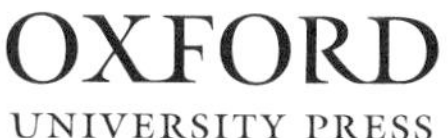

OXFORD
UNIVERSITY PRESS

Great Clarendon Street, Oxford OX2 6DP

Oxford University Press is a department of the University of Oxford.
It furthers the University's objective of excellence in research, scholarship,
and education by publishing worldwide in

Oxford New York

Auckland Cape Town Dar es Salaam Hong Kong Karachi
Kuala Lumpur Madrid Melbourne Mexico City Nairobi
New Delhi Shanghai Taipei Toronto

With offices in

Argentina Austria Brazil Chile Czech Republic France Greece
Guatemala Hungary Italy Japan Poland Portugal Singapore
South Korea Switzerland Thailand Turkey Ukraine Vietnam

Oxford is a registered trade mark of Oxford University Press
in the UK and in certain other countries

Published in the United States
by Oxford University Press Inc., New York

First published 2010

British Library Cataloguing in Publication Data
Data available

Library of Congress Cataloging-in-Publication-Data
Data available

Typeset by Cepha Imaging Private Ltd., Bangalore, India
Printed in China
on acid-free paper through
Asia Pacific Offset

ISBN 978–0–19–922955–0

10 9 8 7 6 5 4 3 2 1

Oxford University Press makes no representation, express or implied, that the drug dosages in this book are correct. Readers must therefore always check the product information and clinical procedures with the most up-to-date published product information and data sheets provided by the manufacturers and the most recent codes of conduct and safety regulations. The authors and publishers do not accept responsibility or legal liability for any errors in the text or for the misuse or misapplication of material in this work. Except where otherwise stated, drug dosages and recommendations are for the non-pregnant adult who is not breastfeeding.

Foreword

Hypertension has been recognized as an important cardiovascular disorder since Korotkoff's invention in 1905 of the auscultatory method for sphygmomanometric measurement of arterial pressure. Since then hypertension has reached pandemic proportions in both the developed and developing nations of the world. The abundant accumulation of knowledge pertaining to hypertensive cardiovascular disease has resulted in a series of comprehensive textbooks that tend to have short shelf-lives because of outdated information. To counter this problem, publishers have gone to the handbook format—short, how-to-books with rapid publication times and frequent updates. Unfortunately, many of these practical books that stress brevity have lacked the depth of knowledge necessary to attract the experienced clinician as well as the physician-in-training; the present handbook of hypertension does not suffer from this defect.

Indeed, this book has an excellent balance of pathophysiologic underpinning and a practical, algorithmic approach to diagnosis, prognosis and treatment. There are numerous illustrations, flow-diagrams, and bullet summaries that integrate information in a useful manner—all with salient but limited references. I am particularly impressed with the detailed investigations for evaluating essential hypertension and diagnosing secondary hypertension, which are included in this book, but frequently given short shrift in standard textbooks. The authors have included up-to-date information on monogenic hypertensive syndromes, special populations, and on optimizing antihypertensive management. There is a novel, concluding chapter, entitled 'Hypertension in the 21st century.' This contains controversial topics dealing with prevention and risk assessment, and the emerging concept of arterial stiffness as an independent determinant of cardiovascular risk. Lastly, there is a glossary of clinical trials that make up a considerable evidence-base for therapeutic decision making. The end product is a well organized handbook that will have a wide readership and satisfy both primary care physicians and specialists with a keen interest in the field of hypertension.

Stanley S. Franklin, MD
Clinical Professor of Medicine
University of California, Irvine
USA

Preface

Over the last 100 years there has been enormous progress in the field of hypertension. However, hypertension remains a condition of paradoxes. We now have simple automated sphygmomanometers, effective antihypertensive drugs, complex risk calculators, and a wealth of trial data telling us whom we should treat and with what. Although this has brought enormous practical benefit for the majority, hypertension remains a common disorder—affecting up to a 1/3 of the adult population, and a major cause of premature morbidity and mortality worldwide. Just when we thought we understood the results of the latest major international trial, another contradictory study is published. Painstaking physiological and genetic research has identified potentially remediable causes of hypertension. However, for the vast majority, the cause remains elusive. Indeed, to borrow a quote from Winston Churchill concerning Russia, essential hypertension remains a 'riddle wrapped in a mystery inside an enigma'.

In writing a book, there is a fine line between producing a lengthy, comprehensive textbook, containing all we ever knew about hypertension, which occupies yards of bookshelves and is rarely opened, and a brief guide that is ultimately too superficial and fails to answer key questions or provide supporting evidence. The aim of this book is to provide a practical, user-friendly guide for those individuals managing hypertensive patients in the 21st century. Although a key feature is brevity, our intention is to provide sufficient depth for even the most experienced clinician, in a clearly laid-out style, and with a wealth of illustrations. The book progresses from our current understanding about the mechanisms of hypertension, through diagnosis, investigations, and management, as well as a review of the current evidence base. Key references are provided, as are practical tips on interpreting specialist investigations and using antihypertensive drugs. We hope the reader will find this a useful and practical book in their routine management of this important and common condition.

Joseph Cheriyan
Carmel M. McEniery
Ian B. Wilkinson

Acknowledgements

We wish to acknowledge the kind foreword by Professor Stanley S. Franklin and for the constructive guidance provided by Professor James Ritter. We would also like to thank Dr Kevin O'Shaughnessy (in particular for his help with the genetics chapter), Dr Khin Swe Myint and Dr Timothy Burton for their help with the illustrations and with the general content of this handbook.

Joseph Cheriyan
Carmel M. McEniery
Ian B. Wilkinson

Contents

Detailed contents

Symbols and abbreviations

🕮	cross reference
🖱	website
↑	increase/d
↓	decrease/d
1°	primary
2°	secondary
>	greater than
<	less than
~	approximately
2D	two-dimensional
3D	three-dimensional
ABPM	ambulatory blood pressure monitoring
ACE	angiotensin-converting enzyme
ACEI	angiotensin-converting enzyme inhibitor
ACTH	adrenocorticotrophic hormone
AF	atrial fibrillation
AGE	advanced glycation end products
ALLHAT	Antihypertensive and Lipid Lowering Treatment to Prevent Heart Attack Trial
ALT	alanine aminotransferase
AME	apparent mineralocorticoid excess
ANA	antinuclear antibodies
ANCA	anti-neutrophilic cytoplasmic antibody
ARA	angiotensin receptor antagonist
ARR	aldosterone:renin ratio
ASCOT	Anglo-Scandinavian Cardiac Outcomes Trial
AST	aspartate aminotranferase
AVS	adrenal vein sampling
BAH	bilateral adrenal hyperplasia
BD	twice a day
BHS	British Hypertension Society
BMI	body mass index
BP	blood pressure
CAH	congenital adrenal hyperplasia
CCA	calcium-channel antagonist

CHD	coronary heart disease
CNS	central nervous system
COX	cyclo-oxygenase
CRP	C-reactive protein
CV	cardiovascular
CVD	cardiovascular disease
CXR	chest X-ray
DASH	Dietary Approaches to Stop Hypertension (trial)
DBP	diastolic blood pressure
DCT	distal convoluted tubule
DHBA	dihydroxybenzylamine
DHP	dihydropyridine
DMSA	dimercaptosuccinic acid
DOC	deoxycorticosterone
DTPA	diethylene triamine pentacetic acid
ECG	electrocardiogram
EDTA	ethylenediamine tetraacetic acid
eGFR	estimated glomerular filtration rate
ENaC	epithelial sodium channel
EPO	Erythropoietin
ESC	European Society of Cardiology
ESH	European Society of Hypertension
ESR	erythrocyte sedimentation rate
ESRD	end-stage renal disease
FBC	full blood count
FDG	F-18 fluorodeoxyglucose
F-DOPA	3,4-dihydroxy-6-fluoro-DL-phenylananine
FMD	fibromuscular dysplasia
GBM	glomerular basement membrane
GFR	glomerular filtration rate
GRA	glucocorticoid remediable aldosteronism
GTN	glyceryl trinitrate
h	hour/s
HCTZ	hydrochlorothiazide
HDL	high-density lipoprotein
HELLP	haemolysis, elevated liver enzymes, and low platelets
HIAA	hydroxyindoleacetic acid
HOCM	hypertrophic obstructive cardiomyopathy

HOT	Hypertension Optimal Treatment (study)
HPLC-EC	high performance liquid chromatography electrochemical
HR	hazard ratio
HYVET	Hypertension in the Very Elderly Trial
IDH	isolated diastolic hypertension
Ig	immunoglobulin
ISH	isolated systolic hypertension
ITU	Intensive Therapy Unit
JBS	Joint British Societies
JNC	Joint National Committee on Prevention, Detection, Evaluation and Treatment of High Blood Pressure
LCH	Langerhans cell histiocytosis
LDH	lactate dehydrogenase
LDL	low-density lipoprotein
LFT	liver function tests
LLA	lipid-lowering arm
LVH	left ventricular hypertrophy,
m	metre/s
MAG	mercapto-acetyl-triglycine
MAOI	monoamine oxidase inhibitor
MAP	mean arterial pressure
MEN	multiple endocrine neoplasia
MI	myocardial infarction
min	Minute/s
MIBG	meta-iodobenzylguanidine
MRI	magnetic resonance imaging
NCCT	NaCL co-transporter
NE	noradrenaline/norepinephrine
NHANES	National Health and Nutrition Examination Survey
NICE	National Institute for Health and Clinical Excellence
NMN	normetanephrine
NNT	number needed to treat
NO	nitric oxide
NSAID	non-steroidal anti-inflammatory drug
OCP	oral contraceptive pill
OD	once a day
PHA2	pseudohypoaldosteronism type II
PIH	pregnancy-induced hypertension
PO	by mouth (per os)

PPIH	proteinuric pregnancy-induced hypertension
PTH	parathyroid hormone
PVR	peripheral vascular resistance
PWV	pulse wave velocity
QDS	4 times a day
RAAS	renin–angiotensin–aldosterone system
RCT	randomized controlled trial
RR	relative risk
s	second/s
SBP	systolic blood pressure
SDH	systolic/diastolic hypertension
SHR	spontaneously hypertensive rats
SIADH	syndrome of inappropriate antidiuretic hormone
SPECT	single photon emission computed tomography
SPRINT	Systolic Blood Pressure Intervention Trial
$t_{1/2}$	half life
TC	total cholesterol
TDS	3 times a day
TED	thromboembolic deterrent
TFT	thyroid function test
TG	triglyceride
TIA	transient ischaemic attack
TOD	target organ damage
TROPHY	Trial of Preventing Hypertension
TSH	thyroid-stimulating hormone
U&Es	urea and electrolytes
USS	ultrasound scan
VEGF	vascular endothelial growth factor
VF	ventricular fibrillation
VMA	vanillylmandelic acid
VT	ventricular tachycardia
WHO	World Health Organization

Chapter 1

Aetiology and pathophysiology

Haemodynamics

Basic haemodynamic concepts

Blood pressure (BP) is the force that the blood exerts on the vessel wall and is continuously varying in arteries due to the intermittent nature of the pump (heart) and elastic recoil of the arterial wall. Besides the simple extremes of pressure, i.e. systolic and diastolic, there are 2 major physiological components of the arterial BP (📖 Fig. 1.1):

- Static or 'steady-state': represented by the mean arterial pressure. The sole determinants of the mean arterial pressure are cardiac output and peripheral vascular resistance (PVR):

  Mean pressure = cardiac output × PVR

- Pulsatile: represented by the pulse pressure (difference between systolic and diastolic BP). The principal determinants of pulse pressure are the stroke volume and the stiffness of the large arteries.

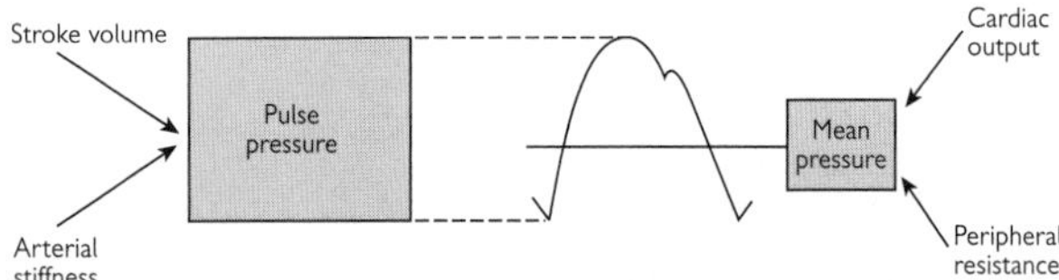

Fig. 1.1 Haemodynamic components of BP. Adapted with permission from Berne RM *et al.* (2004). *Physiology*. Philadelphia, PA: Elsevier, with permission from Elsevier.

Haemodynamics in hypertension

Essential hypertension is characterized by derangements in 1 or more of the physiological determinants of BP mentioned in 🕮 Basic haemodynamic concepts, p.2 although the causal mechanisms remain controversial. Interestingly, age exerts a marked influence on which component becomes abnormal, and this corresponds closely to the form of essential hypertension which is observed (🕮 Fig. 1.2).

Adolescents and young adults (<30 years) with raised BP are often considered to have early, or borderline, hypertension. Here, the principal haemodynamic disturbance is an ↑ stroke volume, whereas PVR is relatively normal. In keeping with this physiological profile, ISH is the predominant form of hypertension observed in young individuals (🕮 Table 1.1).

In contrast, in middle-aged individuals (~30–50 years), cardiac output is normal or even reduced, but the dominant haemodynamic disturbance is a markedly ↑ PVR, which is most likely due to structural remodelling of the resistance vasculature in response to continual exposure to higher pressures. Isolated diastolic hypertension (IDH) or mixed (systolic/diastolic) hypertension (SDH) are the predominant forms of hypertension observed in these individuals. SDH is commonly viewed as the established or 'classical' form of essential hypertension.

In older adults (>50 years), ISH is again the predominant form of hypertension. However, in contrast to the situation in younger individuals, arterial stiffening is the principal haemodynamic disturbance. This causes an exaggerated ↑ in pulse pressure because the large arteries can no longer effectively buffer the cyclical changes in BP during each cardiac cycle.

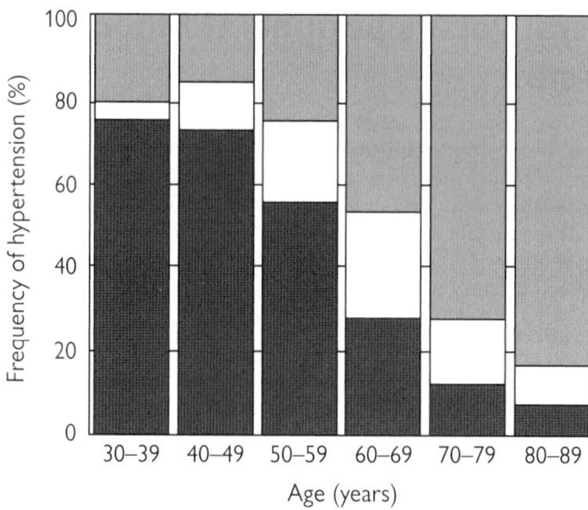

Fig. 1.2 Age-related frequency of different types of hypertension. Data from Sagie A, *et al.* (1993). The natural history of borderline isolated systolic hypertension. *NEJM* **329**:1912–17.

Table 1.1 Age-related haemodynamic patterns underlying hypertension

Age	Principal haemodynamic disturbance	Predominant form of hypertension
<30 years	↑ stroke volume	ISH
30–50 years	↑ PVR	IDH or SDH
>50 years	↑ arterial stiffness	ISH

Central versus peripheral blood pressure

Moving from central (i.e. aorta) to peripheral (i.e. brachial) arteries, systolic pressure ↑ due to differences in vessel stiffness and wave reflections, whereas mean and diastolic pressure fall by only 1–2mmHg (📖 Fig. 1.3). This small fall in mean pressure causes blood to flow forwards, not backwards. The resultant widening or amplification of the pulse pressure—which is more pronounced in younger individuals—means that BP assessed at the brachial artery overestimates BP in the aorta and central arteries.

The difference between brachial and central BP is important because it is the central pressure to which the heart, brain, and other major organs are exposed, and certain drug therapies exert differential effects on peripheral and central pressure. In addition, stratifying individuals by brachial pressure reveals considerable overlap in aortic pressure (📖 Fig. 1.4), which holds important implications for the future categorization of hypertension—if central BP is more important in defining an individual's risk and/or the impact of therapy, then categories that are based on central rather than peripheral pressure may be more useful.

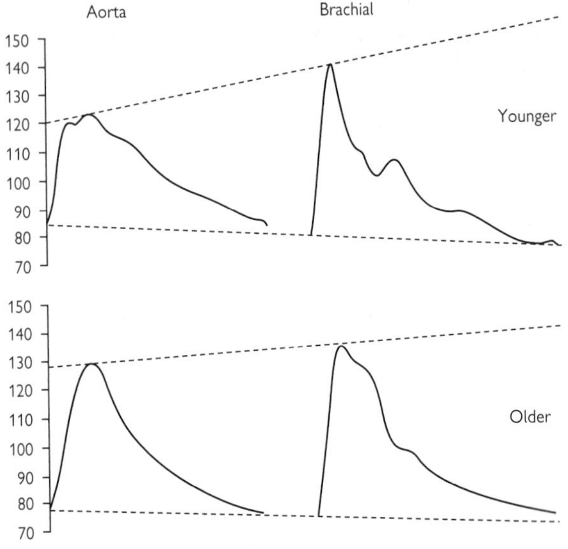

Fig. 1.3 Amplification of BP between central and peripheral arteries.

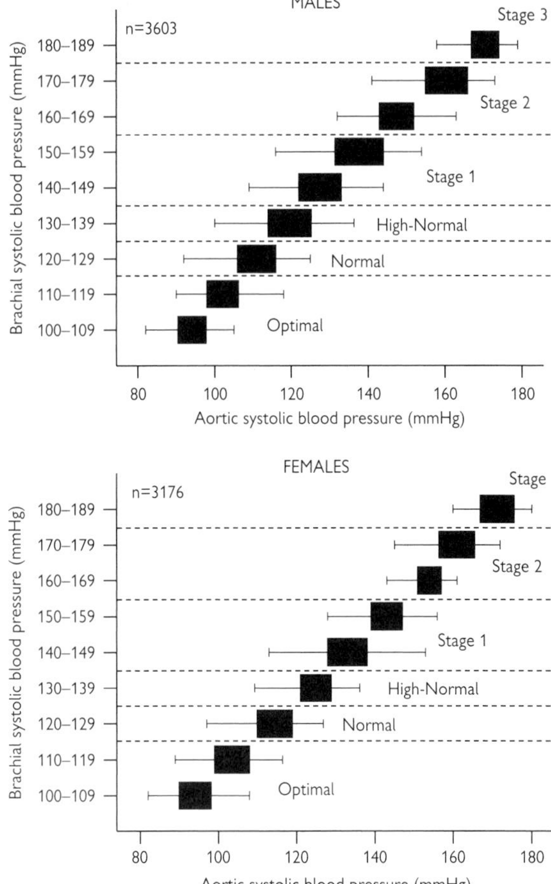

Fig. 1.4 Variation in aortic systolic pressure within categories of brachial systolic pressure. Reproduced with permission from McEniery CM, *et al.* (2008). Central pressure: variability and impact of cardiovascular risk factors. *Hypertension* **51**:1476–82.

Physiology and pathophysiology of blood pressure regulation

The causes underlying the haemodynamic changes observed in essential hypertension remain controversial, although 2 hypotheses predominate. The first is that neurally-mediated factors play a key role in the genesis of raised BP, particularly in young individuals. Evidence of elevated sympathetic nervous system activity (and inactivity of the parasympathetic system) in individuals with mild or borderline essential hypertension includes:

- ↑ resting heart rate.
- ↑ BP response to stimuli such as mental stress, exercise, or the cold pressor test.
- ↑ plasma catecholamine concentrations.

The second major hypothesis explaining the origins of essential hypertension concerns the role of the kidneys and their regulation of the physiological balance between fluid and sodium retention/excretion. Three major renal mechanisms leading to the development of hypertension have been proposed:

- Glomerular filtration rate-dependent mechanisms.
- Transport mechanisms relating to sodium reabsorption.
- Mechanisms relating to renal ischaemia.

The roles of the sympathetic nervous system and renal mechanisms in the physiological and pathophysiological regulation of BP will be discussed in more detail in the rest of this chapter.

Role of the autonomic nervous system

Studies conducted in the 19th century demonstrated that stimulation of peripheral sensory nerves elicited a transient elevation of BP, suggesting that the central nervous system participated in the regulation of BP. Further supporting evidence includes:

- Stressful stimuli (mental arithmetic, cold pressor test) induce a reflex ↑ in BP and heart rate.
- When autonomic drive is lowest (e.g. during sleep) there is a marked reduction in BP and heart rate.

Indeed, tonic discharge from the central nervous system regulates peripheral BP via the release of noradrenaline from sympathetic nerve terminals, acting on adrenergic receptors. In contrast, the parasympathetic nervous system innervates target organs via the release of acetylcholine, acting on muscarinic cholinergic receptors (📖 Fig. 1.5). Overall autonomic activity is determined by the balance between sympathetic and parasympathetic outflow.

Assessment of autonomic nervous system activity

There are a number of methods available to assess autonomic function and the results from a large number of investigations utilizing these methods provide good evidence that ↑ sympathetic nervous system activity is a common feature of individuals with essential hypertension and may even be the initiating mechanism. Individuals exhibiting ↑ sympathetic activity tend to be younger (<40 years), and present with a so-called 'hyperkinetic' state, in which BP, heart rate, and cardiac output are raised—which is not dissimilar to the defence response. Again, this haemodynamic profile is in keeping with the observation that ISH, rather than SDH, is the predominant form of hypertension in younger individuals. Some individuals may also have slightly elevated central arterial stiffness, again possibly due to enhanced sympathetic activation.

Catecholamines (📖 Fig. 1.6)

Plasma and urinary catecholamine concentrations have been used as an index for assessing sympathetic nervous system activity. However, catecholamine concentrations measured in the plasma or urine depend not only on the rate of production and release, but also on the rate of clearance, and, as such, do not provide a very reliable representation of sympathetic nerve activity.

Plasma concentrations of noradrenaline tend to be ↑ in patients with essential hypertension, although the effects are small. Interestingly, acute stress transiently ↑ plasma adrenaline levels and there is some evidence to suggest that mild stressors may cause an exaggerated release of adrenaline in hypertensive subjects whereas no such effects are observed in normotensive individuals. This suggests that individuals with essential hypertension may be more predisposed to the influence of external stressors compared with their normotensive counterparts.

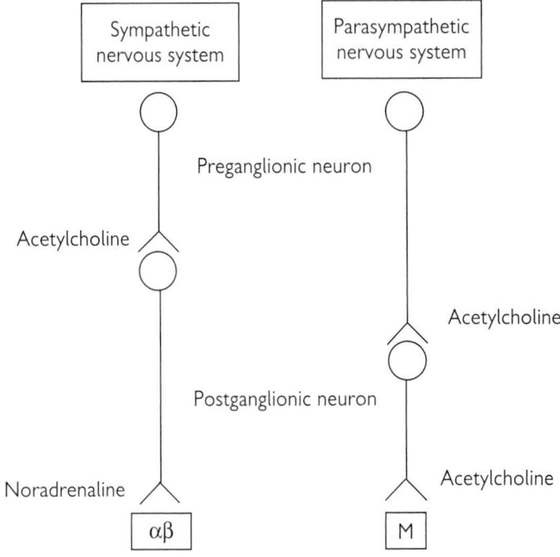

Fig. 1.5 Autonomic nervous system α refers to alpha adrenoceptors; β refers to beta adrenoceptors; M refers to muscarinic cholinergic receptors.

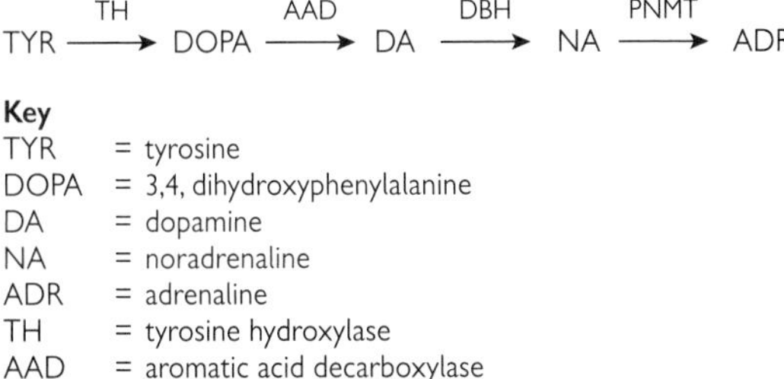

Key

TYR	= tyrosine
DOPA	= 3,4, dihydroxyphenylalanine
DA	= dopamine
NA	= noradrenaline
ADR	= adrenaline
TH	= tyrosine hydroxylase
AAD	= aromatic acid decarboxylase
DBH	= dopamine-β-hydroxylase
PNMT	= phenylethandamine methyltransferase

Fig. 1.6 Biosynthesis of catecholamines.

Noradrenaline spillover

'Spillover studies' measure the rate of noradrenaline entry from sympathetic nerve terminals into plasma and provide a more robust measure of sympathetic nerve activity than measurement of plasma concentrations alone. Tritiated noradrenaline is infused at a constant rate, until a stable arterial concentration is reached, which allows calculation of noradrenaline spillover, clearance, and extraction ratios.

↑ noradrenaline spillover has been observed from the heart and kidneys of hypertensive patients and average total spillover rates are ↑ in patients with essential hypertension up to ~60 years of age. In individuals >60 years, noradrenaline spillover rates tend to be similar to those in normotensive individuals, providing further support for the hypothesis that sympathetic nervous system activity plays an important role in the genesis of hypertension in younger adults.

Microneurography

This technique provides a method of quantifying firing rates in sympathetic nerves. Small electrodes are positioned in subcutaneous sympathetic fibres (typically those of the common peroneal nerve).

The majority of microneurography studies show that nerve firing rates in postganglionic sympathetic fibres passing to skeletal muscle blood vessels are elevated in patients with borderline or mild essential hypertension (📖 Fig. 1.7), and that as hypertension becomes more severe, muscle sympathetic nerve activity ↑ further.

Infusion of adrenergic agonists and antagonists

Adrenergic responsiveness can be assessed by measuring the BP response to a systemic infusion of noradrenaline. However, such responses are affected by endogenous noradrenaline levels, the starting BP and baroreflex sensitivity (📖 see Arterial baroreceptors, p.14). Local (non-systemic) infusions into the brachial artery provide a more precise indication of vascular reactivity. Infusion of adrenergic antagonists can also provide useful information concerning sympathetic activity.

Infusion of propranolol in patients with borderline hypertension reduces cardiac index and heart rate significantly more than in normotensive individuals, indicating ↑ beta-adrenergic drive in patients, although cardiac index and heart rate are not normalized (📖 Fig. 1.8A). However, additional parasympathetic blockade with atropine normalizes cardiac index and heart rate in hypertensives (📖 Fig. 1.8B), although the rise in both indices is less marked, consistent with reduced parasympathetic inhibition.

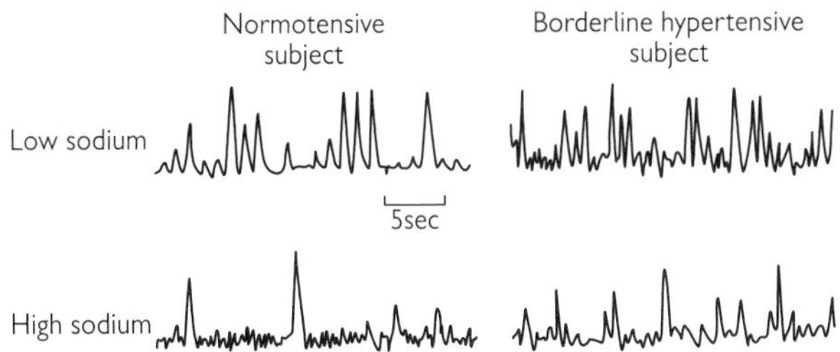

Fig. 1.7 Diagram depicting microneurography tracings. Reproduced with permission from Anderson EA, *et al.* (1989). Elevated sympathetic nerve activity in borderline hypertensive humans. Evidence from direct intraneural recordings. *Hypertension* **14**:177–83.

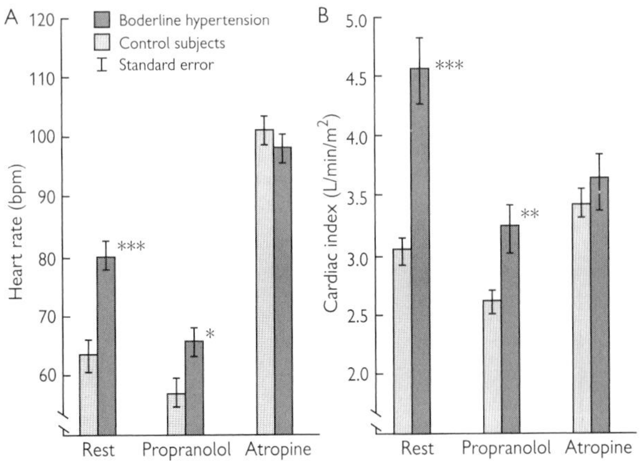

Fig. 1.8 Response to sympathetic and parasympathetic blockade in hypertensives and normotensives. Data from Julius S, *et al.* (1971). Role of parasympathetic inhibition in the hyperkinetic type of borderline hypertension. *Circulation* **44**:413–18.

Spectral analysis of heart rate

Beat-to-beat variability in heart rate is assessed using spectral analysis which yields both low- and high-frequency components of the heart rate variability spectrum. Assessment of high- and low-frequency components of the spectrum allows non-invasive comparison of sympathetic (low-frequency components) and parasympathetic activity (high-frequency components, 📖 see Fig. 1.9). Spectral analysis of heart rate variability indicates that sympathetic components are ↑ and parasympathetic components ↓ in patients with essential hypertension versus normotensive control subjects.

Arterial baroreceptors

Arterial baroreceptors are mechanoreceptors found in the carotid sinus and aortic arch, and the reflexes they initiate provide the major source of short-term regulation of BP by reducing the variability of BP around the prevailing resting value (📖 Fig. 1.10A,B). Peripheral baroreceptor denervation leads to an immediate, marked ↑ in BP and heart rate, which then normalizes, but with ↑ variability. This suggests that the beat-to-beat control of the baroreceptor reflex has been lost but BP remains essentially normal.

Baroreceptor function can be assessed in humans by measuring the response of heart rate to changes in BP—so-called baroreflex sensitivity.

- Hypertensive individuals display reduced baroreflex sensitivity versus normotensive individuals, meaning that for the same ↑ in BP, there is a smaller reduction in heart rate.
- The set point of the baroreceptor reflex (the point at which alterations in BP will trigger alterations in sympathetic tone) operates at a higher BP in hypertensive subjects and operates across a narrower range of BPs with ↑ severity of hypertension.

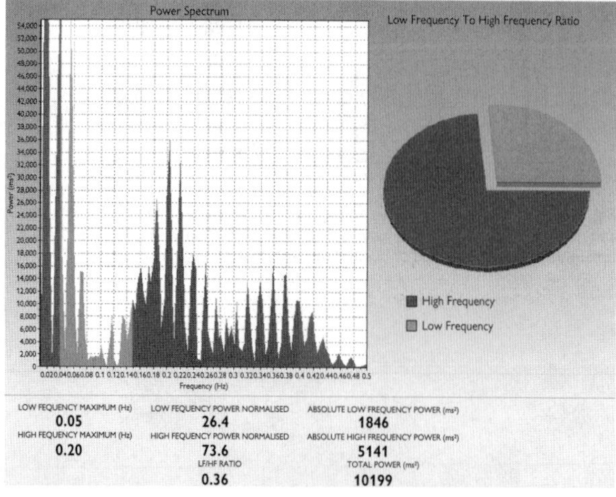

Fig. 1.9 Spectral analysis of heart rate variability. High frequency components ■ indicate parasympathetic activity; low frequency components ■ indicate sympathetic activity.

A

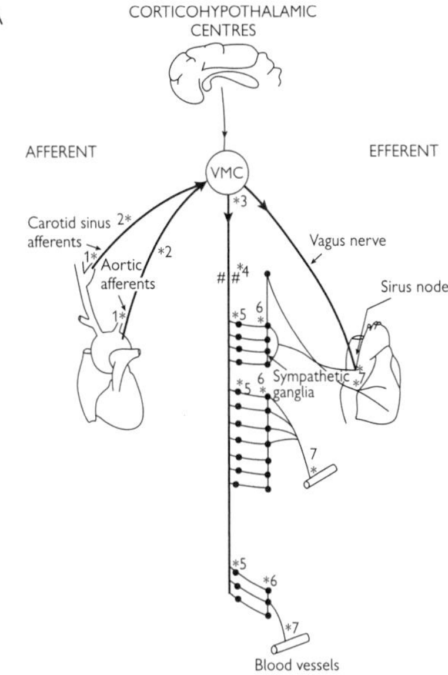

B

Arterial BP level	Low	Normal	High
Carotid sinus nerve (no. impulses)	+	++	+++
Vagus nerve (no. impulses)	+	++	+++
Sympathetic cardiac nerve (no. impulses)	+++	++	+
Sympathetic vasoconstrictor nerve (no. impulses)	+++	++	+

Fig. 1.10 Afferent and autonomic efferent pathways of the baroreflex arc. Adapted from Mathias CJ and Banister R (2001). *Autonomic failure: a textbook of clinical disorders of the autonomic nervous system,* Oxford University Press.

Role of the kidneys

The kidneys play a major role in the physiological control of BP through the regulation of sodium and fluid balance. The renin–angiotensin system is a key component of this regulation. However, whether the kidneys contribute to the initiation of essential hypertension is somewhat controversial.

Renin–angiotensin–aldosterone system (RAAS)

A major physiological role of the RAAS is to maintain BP in situations where renal blood flow or blood volume is reduced (📖 Fig. 1.11). Therefore, in healthy, well-hydrated individuals, this system is relatively inactive. However:

- Elevated renin levels have been observed in some individuals with essential hypertension, suggesting that the RAAS may cause the elevated BP in these individuals.
- Effective BP control can be achieved in some hypertensive individuals by blocking the effects of the RAAS using beta-blockers, angiotensin converting enzyme (ACE) inhibitors, or angiotensin receptor antagonists (ARAs).

Therefore, the RAAS is actively involved in at least some individuals with essential hypertension although the precise role of the renin–angiotensin system in the genesis of essential hypertension more generally is controversial. The RAAS does, however, play an important role in secondary forms of hypertension due to renal artery stenosis (RAS) (📖 see Renal artery stenosis, p.138), or rare monogenic syndromes (📖 see Chapter 5 p.169).

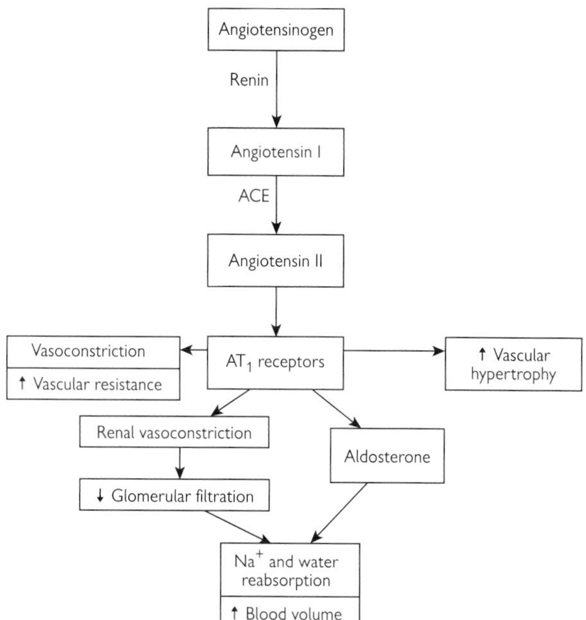

Fig. 1.11 The renin–angiotensin–aldosterone system. Adapted from Wilkins R, *et al.* (2006). *Oxford Handbook of Medical Sciences*. Oxford: Oxford University Press, with permission from Oxford University Press.

Guyton's theory of hypertension

Salt intake and renal sodium handling form the basis of Guyton's theory on the long-term control of BP, which he developed nearly 40 years ago with the use of mathematical modelling and computer programming. He largely ignored the role of the autonomic nervous system and argued that it was the kidneys which were of key importance in determining the arterial pressure. According to Guyton, all forms of hypertension are caused by a chronic excess of salt intake. Therefore:

- Individuals who develop hypertension have abnormal renal function causing fluid and sodium imbalances as a direct result of excessive sodium intake. BP then becomes elevated, leading to the development of sustained hypertension (📖 Fig. 1.12).
- Individuals who remain normotensive in the face of excessive sodium intake have preserved renal function, allowing rapid restoration of fluid and sodium imbalances before BP starts to rise.

The major problem with Guyton's hypothesis was that the experimental evidence did not fully support the predictions of his model. Dogs with surgically reduced renal mass developed sustained hypertension which was accompanied by an ↑ cardiac output related to volume overload, but a gradual and unexpected rise in PVR was also observed. To explain the unanticipated rise in PVR, Guyton devised the concept of 'long-term autoregulation' where an ↑ PVR results from adjustments in vascular tone occurring after a long latency. However, in contrast to Guyton's theory, not all forms of hypertension exhibit this haemodynamic pattern. Moreover, this pattern is most typical of early, borderline hypertension where, ironically, sympathetic nervous system activation contributes to an elevated cardiac output and then structural remodelling contributes to the later rise in PVR.

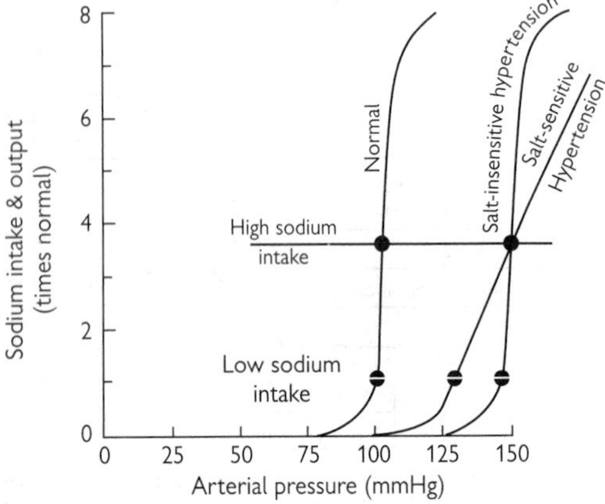

Fig. 1.12 Shift of the renal function curve from normotensive levels to hypertensive levels, as postulated by Guyton. Redrawn with permission, from the *Annual Review of Medicine*, vol. 31, ©1980 Annual Reviews, http://www.annualreviews.org

Renal mechanisms leading to essential hypertension

Despite the flaws in Guyton's theory, additional lines of evidence suggest that the kidneys may indeed play a role in pathogenesis of hypertension:

- Hypertension is a common feature of renal disease.
- BP correlates with sodium intake and can be improved with sodium restriction.
- Transplant studies in animals and humans have demonstrated that kidneys from hypertensive donors ↑ BP in normotensive recipients. Conversely, kidneys from normotensive donors lower BP in hypertensive recipients.

Several mechanisms have been proposed:

- Glomerular filtration rate (GFR)-dependent mechanisms:
  - ↓GFR may lead to sodium retention and volume expansion.
  - Animal models with removed or injured kidneys develop hypertension rapidly.

- In humans, the frequency of hypertension ↑ with ↓GFR. However, with normal kidney function, a reduced rate of filtering should be counterbalanced by reduced sodium reabsorption, implying that the development of hypertension depends upon some degree of impaired renal tubular sodium handling. This mechanism probably underlies hypertension in renal disease, diabetes, and, in some cases, ageing. However, in most cases of essential hypertension, GFR is normal or only minimally depressed.

- Transport mechanisms related to sodium reabsorption:
  - Since the collecting ducts of the nephron are key to the final regulation of sodium excretion/reabsorption, impaired regulation of sodium transport in the collecting ducts may result in impaired sodium excretion. The primary action of aldosterone is to ↑ sodium reabsorption in the collecting ducts and, apart from being secreted by tumours, aldosterone may also be involved in a number of forms of low renin hypertension, such as obesity. Certain oxidized fatty acids can stimulate aldosterone production and levels of both are raised in some obese individuals with essential hypertension.
- Renal ischaemia:
  - Renal vasoconstriction, most likely at the afferent arteriole, is mediated by a number of mechanisms including oxidative stress, angiotensin II, and nitric oxide (NO) deficiency. Evidence of mild tubular ischaemia and inflammation has been observed in hypertensive patients, leading to more severe renal arteriolar disease over time. Two phases are likely to occur: (1) agents causing systemic and intrarenal vasoconstriction, such as endothelial-derived mediators, activation of the RAAS, and overactivity of the sympathetic nervous system which cause the onset of hypertension; (2) renal microvascular disease and infiltration of inflammatory cells serves to prolong renal vasoconstriction, predisposing to vascular remodelling.

Interplay between autonomic and renal mechanisms

The evidence from renal transplant studies in animals suggests that essential hypertension is caused by a genetic or developmental renal fault, thus prompting Dahl to utter his famous dictum 'blood pressure travels with the kidneys'.[1] However, the majority of patients with essential hypertension exhibit normal renal function, at least initially, suggesting that non-renal mechanisms are probably responsible for the genesis of essential hypertension, whereas renal mechanisms contribute to the sustained nature of this condition. In contrast, resting sympathetic nervous system activity is elevated in individuals with borderline essential hypertension and this probably explains the initiation of most forms of essential hypertension, at least in younger individuals. Interestingly, sympathetic nervous system activation stimulates the RAAS, providing an important link between the autonomic nervous system and the kidney (📖 Fig. 1.13).

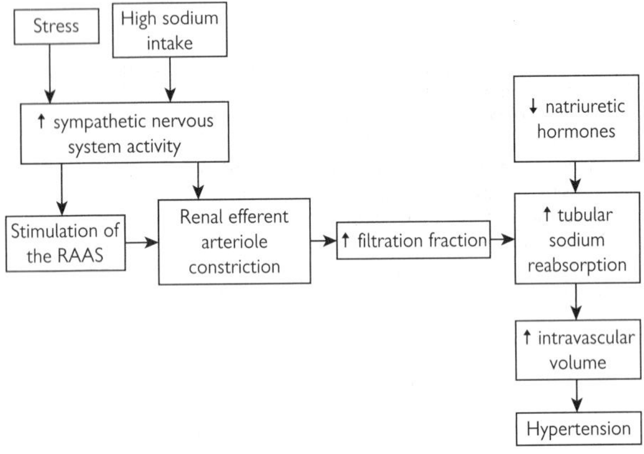

Fig. 1.13 Interplay between the sympathetic nervous system and renal mechanisms in the development of essential hypertension. Adapted from Kaplan NM (1988). Systemic hypertension: mechanisms and diagnosis. In Braunwald E (ed) *Heart Disease*, pp.819–83. Philadelphia, PA: WB Saunders, with permission from Elsevier.

Reference

1. Dahl LK, Heine M, Thompson K. (1974). Genetic influence of the kidneys on blood pressure. *Circulation Research*, **34**:94–101.

Vascular structure and function in essential hypertension

Although neural, humoral, and haemodynamic factors appear to initiate the development of essential hypertension in younger individuals, continual exposure to elevated BP leads to a number of structural and functional adaptations within the resistance vasculature. Such changes result in sustained ↑ in BP which, once initiated, are largely irreversible. In contrast, in older individuals, ↑ large artery stiffness directly contributes to the rise in systolic and pulse pressure observed in these individuals.

Structural changes in resistance vessels

Poisseuille's law states that the resistance of a vessel is inversely proportional to the fourth power of the vessel radius. Therefore, even small reductions in vessel diameter will have a large effect on the vascular resistance to blood flow. In established 'classical' essential hypertension, the walls of resistance vessels are characterized by thickening and/or remodelling of the media, leading to a reduction in lumen diameter and an ↑ wall:lumen ratio. This adaptation contributes significantly to the ↑ in vascular resistance which is a dominant feature of 'classical' essential hypertension. Two major mechanisms account for the reduction in lumen diameter (📖 Fig. 1.14):

- Hypertrophic remodelling: pressure-induced ↑ in medial mass associated with smooth muscle cell hypertrophy and also an ↑ in connective tissue, such as collagen.
- Eutrophic remodelling: vessel wall remodelling leading to a reduction in lumen diameter, but no overall growth of cellular or connective tissue. This form of remodelling appears to arise from hypertrophic remodelling. The vessel wall is then subject to apoptosis in the outer medial layer and fibrosis of the adventitia, which prevents further ↑ in wall mass.

A further structural change in hypertensive resistance vessels is rarefaction (closure/loss of arterioles) as a consequence of sustained vasoconstriction. Rarefaction is mostly transient although individuals with mild to moderate essential hypertension exhibit longer periods of rarefaction compared with normotensive individuals. Vessel rarefaction reduces the total cross-sectional area of the resistance vasculature and thus contributes to the rise in PVR.

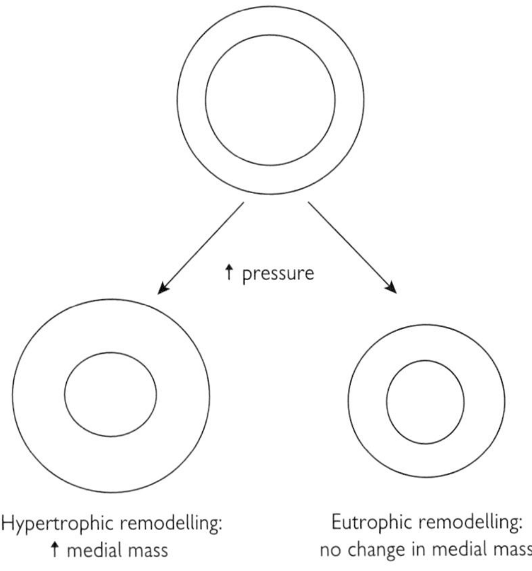

Fig. 1.14 Resistance vessel remodelling in response to high BP.

Functional changes in resistance vessels

Increased sensitivity to vasoconstrictors

↑ sensitivity to vasoconstrictor substances has been observed in hypertensive individuals although the precise mechanisms are controversial. The ↑ sensitivity could be a result of ↑ receptor sensitivity or activation of second messenger pathways. Alternatively, structural adaptations within the arterial wall, such as smooth muscle hypertrophy or ↑ wall: lumen ratios result in ↑ force generation for a given concentration of vasoconstrictor.

Endothelial dysfunction

A number of, but not all, studies suggest that endothelium-dependent vasodilatation is impaired in essential hypertension. Possible mechanisms for this impairment include reduced production/release of NO, a potent vasodilator molecule, ↑ degradation of NO by free radicals, or an imbalance in the production of endothelium-derived vasodilatory factors versus vasoconstrictor factors (such as endothelin). In addition, the vascular smooth muscle may exhibit reduced responsiveness to vasodilators such as NO, although this is not thought to be a major mechanism underlying impaired dilatory responses observed in hypertensive individuals.

Structural changes develop gradually as essential hypertension progresses. These changes enhance vasoconstrictor responses and ↑ the degree of rarefaction, further ↑ BP. A probable initiating mechanism for these structural changes is sympathetic nervous system activation, which can remain elevated for a number of years. The structural and functional abnormalities listed earlier in this section then assume a dominant role in maintaining the elevated BP. Once initiated, this process is largely irreversible (📖 Fig. 1.15).

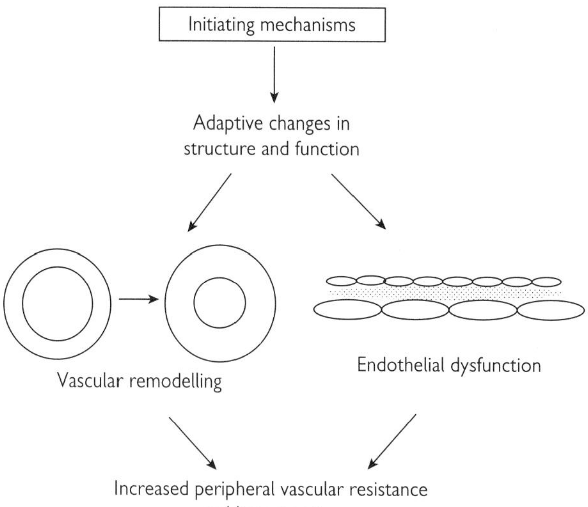

Fig. 1.15 Vascular mechanisms underlying 'classical' essential hypertension.

Large arteries

Large arteries were once considered as inert conduits, but are now recognized to play an important physiological role in buffering the oscillatory changes in BP resulting from intermittent ventricular ejection. This action reduces pulse pressure, smoothes peripheral blood flow, and improves the efficiency of the cardiovascular (CV) system as a whole. However, stiffening of large arteries leads to a number of adverse haemodynamic consequences, and may promote disease by a number of different mechanisms including:

- Widening of pulse pressure i.e. ↑ systolic BP (SBP)/↓ diastolic BP (DBP) leading to:
  - ISH.
  - Left ventricular hypertrophy (LVH) and ventricular stiffening, leading to diastolic dysfunction and heart failure (↑ SBP).
  - Reduction in diastolic pressure, leading to a reduction in coronary blood flow, predisposing to ischaemia (↓ DBP).
- ↑ cyclical stress on arterial walls leading to accelerated elastic fibre fatigue fracture which causes further ↑ in arterial stiffness.
- Transmission of pulsatile stress to other large arteries e.g. carotid, leading to wall remodelling and intima-media thickening.
- Transmission of pulsatile stress to microvascular beds of the brain and kidney.
- ↓ shear stress rate leading to ↓ endothelial NO production (a key event in atheroma formation).

Structural changes in large arteries

The large arteries undergo a number of age-related structural changes within the arterial wall. One of the most consistent structural changes is the gradual dilatation and hardening of the arteries (arteriosclerosis). This is partly the result of fatigue fracture of the elastic elements within the medial layer, and often considered a consequence of 'wear and tear' on the arteries. Indeed, by the age of 60 years, the average individual will have experienced >2 billion stress cycles of the aorta (average heart rate × age). The ↑ pulse pressure which results from this process exerts an additive stress on the arterial wall, further ↑ cyclical stress and setting up a vicious cycle.

Other structural changes occurring in large arteries include ↑ collagen deposition and, therefore, alterations in the ratio of elastin, collagen, and other matrix proteins. There is also an ↑ formation of advanced glycation end products (AGEs), which are a heterogeneous group of protein and lipids to which sugar residues are covalently bound, and which accumulate slowly on long-lived matrix proteins such as elastin and collagen. Finally, calcification of the medial layer occurs with ↑ frequency in older individuals and contributes to the ↑ rate of arterial stiffening observed in older individuals (📖 Fig. 1.16).

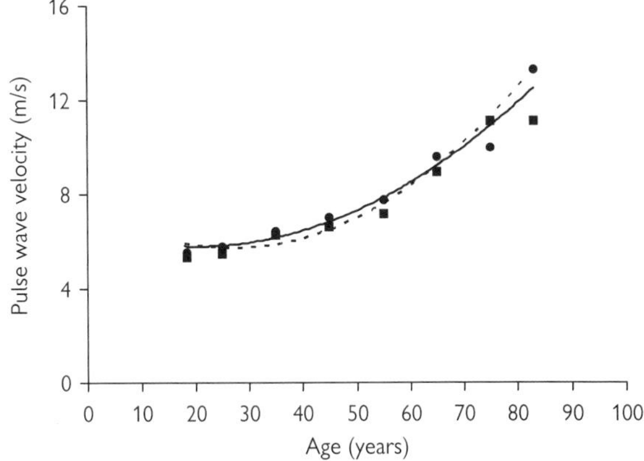

Fig. 1.16 The effect of age on aortic pulse wave velocity (squares = women; circles = men). Reproduced from McEniery CM, *et al.* (2005). Normal vascular aging: differential effects on wave reflection and aortic pulse wave velocity: The Anglo-Cardiff Collaborative Trial (ACCT). *J Am Coll Cardiol* **46**:1753–60, with permission from Elsevier.

Genetics of essential hypertension

It has often been stated that ~40% of hypertension is attributable to genetic influences. However, although specific genetic variants might determine who is susceptible to the development of hypertension, environmental factors also exert significant effects on BP, making it difficult to distinguish between genetic and environmental influences. Overall, genetic factors are thought to result in ↑ BP when interacting with *permissible* environmental factors.

Essential hypertension is a complex condition and, as yet, there is a relatively poor understanding of the genetic pathways involved in the development of this condition. To date, only rare monogenic mutations which share a relationship with altered salt homeostasis have been conclusively identified as causes of hypertension (📖 see Monogenic syndromes, p.169).

Problems in understanding the genetic basis of essential hypertension

Essential hypertension is physiologically complex

A large number of haemodynamic and biochemical mechanisms potentially lead to the development of essential hypertension, making it a physiologically complex condition. Therefore, it is not surprising that the genetic basis of hypertension is similarly complex. Animal models of hypertension have aided our understanding of certain physiological and biochemical mechanisms, but although these models mimic essential hypertension, they do not necessarily represent the true situation in humans *in vivo*.

Essential hypertension is phenotypically complex

Essential hypertension has a number of different forms, arising from distinct haemodynamic and pathophysiological mechanisms (📖 see Haemodynamics in hypertension, p.4). However, many of the large-scale genetic association studies conducted to date have treated hypertension as a single, uniform condition, which reduces the likelihood of identifying specific causative genes. Improving the way in which we define sub-types of essential hypertension will be a key factor in advancing our understanding of its genetic causes.

Essential hypertension is associated with significant genetic heterogeneity

BP is a continuous parameter and such parameters are usually polygenic (the product of many genes). Therefore, the development of essential hypertension probably reflects the small, additive effects of many genes. Indeed, finding individual gene variants with a measurable effect on BP has been difficult. It is also likely that different subsets of genes influence BP in different people and yet the end product (raised BP) appears to be similar across a large number of individuals.

Major approaches to studying the genetics of essential hypertension

Genetic linkage analysis

Many physical traits tend to be genetically transmitted together, from 1 generation to the next—a process termed genetic linkage. It is this phenomenon which forms the basis for gene identification in large families (pedigrees) with multiple generations (family-based linkage) and in populations (linkage disequilibrium mapping). Linkage analysis allows the identification of numerous chromosomal regions which are likely to harbour genetic variants influencing BP. If small enough regions are isolated, then specific genes and their variants can be identified using gene sequencing methods. This approach has been successful in identifying the mutated genes responsible for monogenic forms of hypertension. However, due to the vast genetic and phenotypic heterogeneity associated with essential hypertension, linkage analysis has provided little insight into the genetic basis of this condition.

Gene association studies

In these studies, genetic and phenotypic variation is compared using a case–control design. Therefore, variants of specific genes are compared between hypertensive and normotensive individuals, an approach which requires careful matching for potentially confounding factors such as age, gender, and race. Recent developments in high throughput genotyping and statistical methods for analysing large amounts of genetic data should theoretically allow whole-genome association studies. This is based upon the principle that by identifying enough genetic variants in a large number of individuals with different hypertensive phenotypes, it will be possible to examine every gene for an association with BP variation and to identify a set of genes which are responsible for influencing BP regulation. However, at present, this approach is effort intensive and prohibitively expensive.

Genetic mapping

This approach involves genotyping individuals from different populations (i.e. with different geographic origins) in order to create a common map of the human genome—a strategy which has been adopted by the Hapmap project, which has been designed to provide a catalogue of common genetic variants occurring within humans. The genome is made up of a mosaic of blocks of deoxyribonucleic acid (DNA) spanning intervals between recombination sites. Most of the DNA sequence within blocks is the same between individuals, meaning that these blocks can be characterized by small sets of sites that differ—single nucleotide polymorphisms (SNPs). Certain sets of SNPs tend to be inherited together and these regions of linked SNPs are known as haplotypes. Ultimately, it may be possible to identify blocks of DNA containing the genes associated with essential hypertension by comparing the distribution of haplotypes between hypertensive and normotensive individuals.

Future of genetic studies in hypertension

Despite the obvious challenges associated with examining the genetics of hypertension, recent advances in technology are likely to improve understanding of the specific gene variants contributing to this condition. A long-term aim of genetic studies will be to utilize information such as that provided by the Hapmap project, to predict the development of hypertension before signs of the disease appear. Ultimately such an approach may allow us to prevent the onset of this condition. There is also a great deal of interest in pharmacogenetics—the identification of genes which influence an individual's response to pharmacologic therapy, which may allow treatment to be tailored more appropriately to individual requirements.

Environmental influences on blood pressure

In almost all societies worldwide, there are marked changes in BP with age (📖 Fig. 1.17):

- SBP rises throughout life—indeed, this appears to be accelerated after the age of ~50 years.
- DBP rises until ~50 years of age and then plateaus, or even declines.
- Pulse pressure ↑, especially after ~50 years of age.

Although such changes in BP were once considered to be inevitable, several lines of evidence suggest that this is not the case:

- The age-related changes in BP are absent or greatly reduced in a number of rural populations, including Easter Islanders, Soloman Islanders, Highlanders of Papua New Guinea, African Bushmen, and Zulu tribes (📖 Fig. 1.18).
- Migration of the inhabitants of rural-dwelling communities to industrialized areas results in a steeper age-related rise in BP (📖 Fig. 1.19).

These observations suggest that whilst genetic influences on BP are important, lifestyle factors such as diet, physical activity level, and stress exert a major influence on BP.

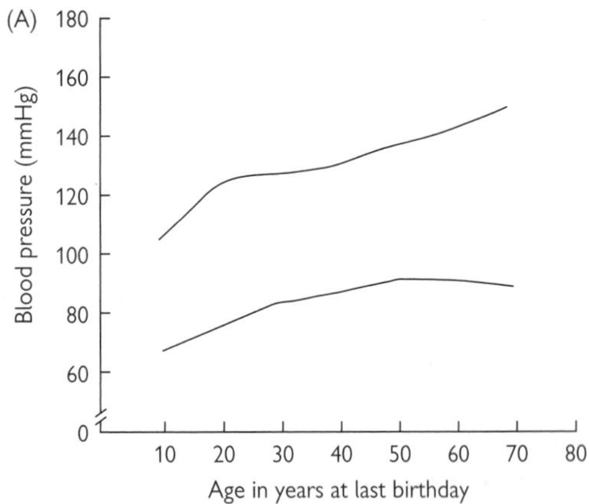

Fig. 1.17 Changes in BP with age. Data from Burt V, *et al.* (1995). Prevalence of hypertension in the US adult population: results from the Third National Health and Nutrition Examination Survey, 1988–1991. *Hypertension* **25**:305–13.

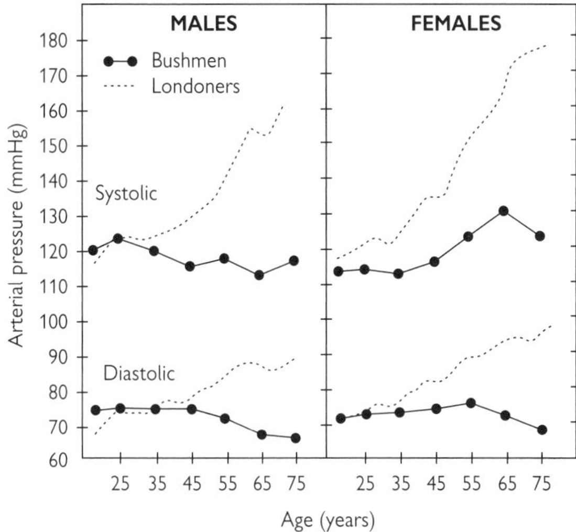

Fig. 1.18 Influence of age on BP in Kung Bushmen in Northern Botswana, compared with people from London, UK ('Londoners'). Reproduced from Truswell AS, *et al.* (1972). Blood pressures of Kung bushmen in Northern Botswana. *Am Heart J* **84**:5–12, with permission from Elsevier.

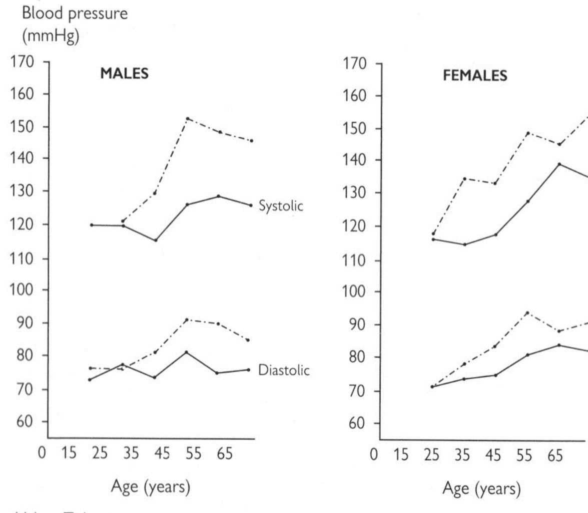

Fig. 1.19 Influence of age on systolic and diastolic BP in rural and urban Zulus compared to the black and white populations of Georgia, USA. Adapted with permission from Scotch NA, *et al.* (1963). Sociocultural factors in the epidemiology of Zulu hypertension. *Am J Public Health* **53**:1205–13, © American Public Health Association.

Physical activity

Evidence from epidemiological studies shows an inverse relationship between the amount of physical activity undertaken and level of BP, although many of the studies did not control for other factors associated with hypertension, between active and inactive groups. However, evidence from a recent meta-analysis demonstrates that regular aerobic exercise (rhythmic endurance exercise involving large muscle groups) can lower SBP by 2–7mmHg, with the greatest fall in BP observed in hypertensive patients (📖 Fig. 1.20). Resistance training may also be beneficial in lowering BP (reported fall in SBP between 3–6mmHg) although fewer studies have investigated the antihypertensive effects of this form of exercise. Indeed, resistance training is most likely to have beneficial effects as part of an overall fitness regimen, but is not recommended as a sole form of exercise. Current guidelines recommend aerobic exercise such as brisk walking for >30min per day at a moderate intensity, equating to ~50–70% of an individual's maximum heart rate (220 minus age).

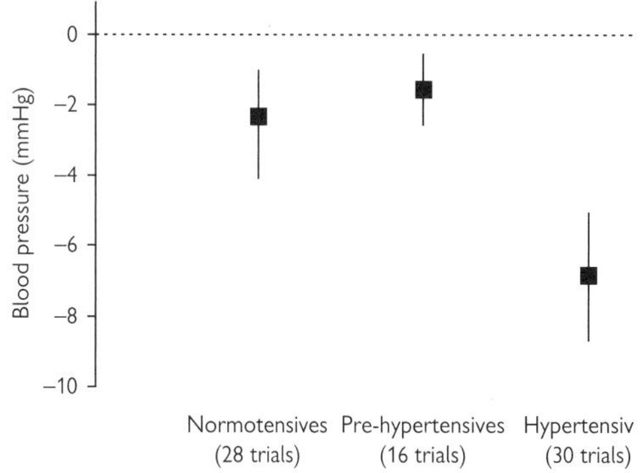

Fig. 1.20 Results of meta-analysis of 74 randomized controlled trials testing the effects of aerobic exercise on BP. Based on data from Cornelisson VA, *et al.* (2005). Effects of endurance training on blood pressure, blood pressure–regulating mechanisms, and cardiovascular risk factors. *Hypertension* **46**:667–5.

Diet

Interaction between sodium and potassium intake

For many years, sodium has been considered to be the most influential dietary factor in the development of essential hypertension. However, the role of potassium should not be overlooked. Indeed, rather than considering the roles of sodium and potassium in isolation, recent attention has focused on the interplay between these factors as being the most important dietary cause of elevated BP.

Physiologically, humans are adapted to retain salt and lose potassium, a mechanism which is largely due to the diets of early humans which were low in salt and rich in potassium. However, the diets of individuals living in modern, industrialized societies tend to be high in sodium and low in potassium, which requires the kidneys to excrete excess sodium and retain potassium. A failure of the kidneys to adapt to and compensate for the modern, westernized diet results in an excess of retained sodium and a deficit in potassium, leading ultimately to vascular smooth muscle contraction, ↑ PVR, and, ultimately, elevated BP (📖 Fig. 1.21).

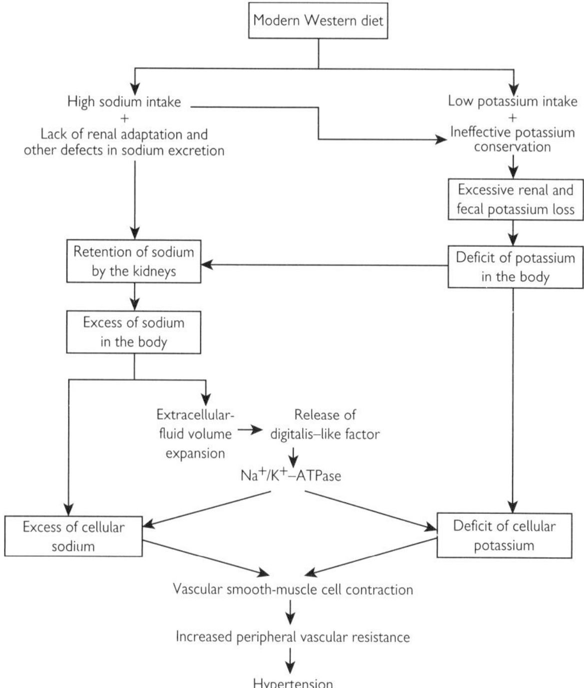

Fig. 1.21 Interaction between sodium and potassium intake in the pathogenesis of essential hypertension. Reproduced with permission from Adrogue HJ and Madias NE (2007). Sodium and potassium in the pathogenesis of hypertension. *NEJM* **356**:1966–78.

Salt intake

Physiologically, the daily requirement for salt is ~8–10mmol/day and early humans probably consumed ~20–40mmol/day. However, the average daily salt intake of individuals living in industrialized societies is ~140–150mmol/day—10–20 times the physiological requirement—which then must be excreted by the kidneys. Numerous studies suggest a positive association between salt intake and BP. However, the best evidence of a direct relationship between the level of salt intake and level of BP comes from the Intersalt study[1] in which salt intake and BP levels were assessed in over 10,000 individuals from 32 countries. Salt intake was determined by 24-h urinary sodium concentrations. A strong positive association between sodium excretion and BP was observed, suggesting that salt intake does indeed influence BP level (📖 Fig. 1.22).

Further studies have confirmed and extended the findings of the Intersalt study by demonstrating that a reduction in the level of salt intake results in lower BP. The best evidence comes from the DASH study diet[2], which is high in fresh fruit and vegetables, and low in sodium and dairy products. The study was conducted in patients with borderline hypertension and a reduction in BP was observed after 4 weeks on the diet. In a follow-up study (DASH-sodium)[3], 3 levels of sodium intake were included and a dose–response relationship was observed between the level of sodium restriction and the extent of reduction in BP. Taken together, these observations suggest a very potent relationship between salt intake and BP. However, a firm link between a reduction in sodium intake and a concomitant reduction in CV events has not yet been observed.

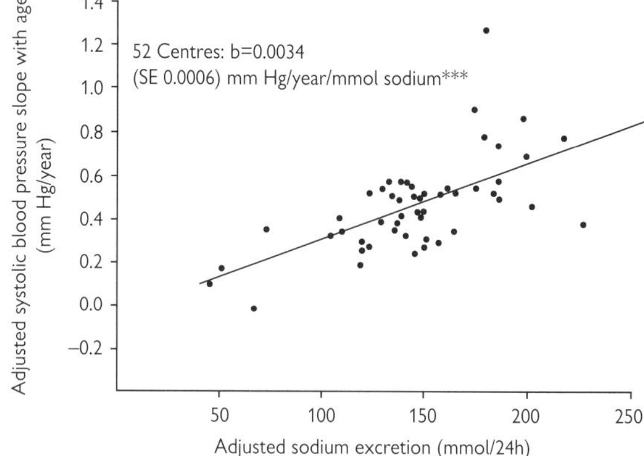

Fig. 1.22 Relationship between sodium excretion and systolic BP in the Intersalt study. Reproduced from Intersalt Cooperative Research Group (1988). Intersalt: an international study of electrolyte excretion and blood pressure. Results for 24-hour urinary sodium and potassium excretion. *BMJ* **297**:319–28. Copyright © 1988, with permission from BMJ Publishing Group.

References

1. INTERSALT Cooperative Research Group (1988). INTERSALT: an international study of electrolyte excretion and blood pressure. Results for 24 hour urinary sodium and potassium excretion. *BMJ* **297**:319–28.
2. Appel LJ, Moore TJ, Obarzanek E, *et al.* (1997). A clinical trail of the effects of dietary patterns on blood pressure. *NEJM*, **336**:1117–24.
3. Sacks FM, Svetkey LP, Volmer WM, Appel LJ, *et al.* (2001). Effects on blood pressure of reduced dietary sodium and the dietary approaches to stop hypertension (DASH) Diet. *NEJM*, **344**:3–10.

Potassium intake

Epidemiological data suggest an inverse association between potassium intake and BP, since in rural-based populations where the typical diet is rich in potassium, the age-related ↑ in BP is far less marked than urban populations. However, the Intersalt study provided firm evidence of an inverse association between potassium intake and the level of BP, where a 50mmol/day ↑ in urinary potassium excretion was associated with a 3.4mmHg ↓ in SBP and 1.9mmHg ↓ in DBP. Clinical trials have provided further evidence that ↑ potassium intake results in ↓ BP. A meta-analysis of 33 randomized controlled trials in >2500 hypertensive and normotensive subjects showed that overall, an ↑ intake of potassium was associated with reductions in SBP of ~4% and in DBP of 2.5%, with a larger effect on BP observed in HT subjects. The precise mechanism by which ↑ potassium intake exerts an anti-hypertensive effect remains unclear. Proposed mechanisms include a direct natriuretic effect, suppression of the RAAS system and the sympathetic nervous system, and a direct arterial vasodilatory effect (Fig. 1.23).

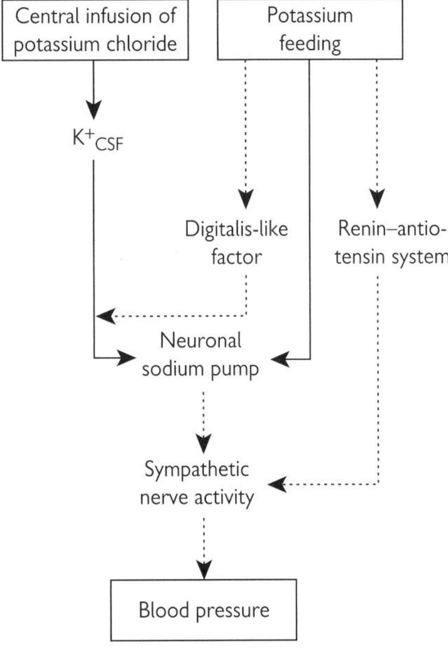

Fig. 1.23 Central effects of potassium infusion or potassium feeding on the BP of normotensive rats. Solid lines indicate an increase, broken lines indicate a decrease or inhibition. Reproduced with permission from Adrogue HJ and Madias NE (2007). Sodium and potassium in the pathogenesis of hypertension. *NEJM* **356**:1966–78.

Alcohol

Despite some evidence demonstrating that the relationship between alcohol intake and BP is J-shaped, overall, there is a positive association between BP and alcohol intake in both men and women. Moreover, the risk associated with alcohol consumption ↑ beyond moderate levels of intake. Acute and chronic alcohol consumption causes a rise in BP, and a recent meta-analysis reports that a reduction in alcohol intake reduces SBP and DBP by 3 and 2 mm Hg respectively. In hypertensive patients, reductions in SBP (5–8mmHg) and DBP (2–3mmHg) have been reported. A reduction in alcohol consumption is also associated with weight loss which probably aids in the BP-lowering effect. Current recommendations are that hypertensive patients should drink less than 2 units of alcohol per day.

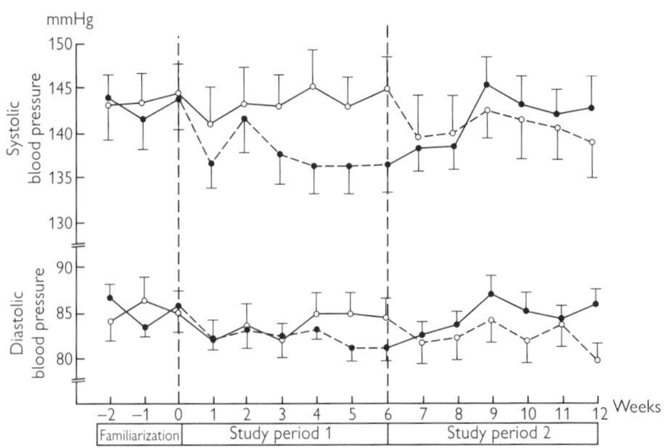

Fig. 1.24 Effect of reduction in alcohol intake on blood pressure. Reproduced from Puddy I, *et al.* (1987). Regular alcohol use raises blood pressure in treated hypertensive subjects: a randomized control trial. *Lancet.* **329**:647–51. © 1987 with permission from Elsevier.

Reference

1. Xin X *et al.* (2001). Effects of alcohol reduction on blood pressure. A meta-analysis of randomised clinical trails. *Hypertension.* **38**: 1112–17.

Stress

Acute and chronic exposure to emotional stress will elevate BP in virtually all individuals, but BP tends to normalize when the stressful period ends. Therefore, the precise role of stress in the genesis of essential hypertension is unclear. Nevertheless, cross-sectional and longitudinal evidence suggests that stress is an important environmental factor which contributes to ↑ in BP.

Cross-sectional evidence

- Acute ↑ in stress induced by laboratory procedures (mental stress tests, mental arithmetic) is matched by acute ↑ in BP.
- In individuals of a given socio-economic status, BPs are higher in those who live and/or work in stressful environments than those in less stressful environments.

Longitudinal evidence

- In a classic observational study, age-related changes in BP were compared between a community of nuns living in secluded orders and age-matched women (many of whom were relatives) living in urbanized society within a similar geographic region.[1] Despite similar dietary and, in particular, sodium levels between the participants, the nuns exhibited markedly lower BPs at all ages. The routine, quiet lifestyle led by the nuns suggested that the major difference between the groups was the level of chronic stress encountered (📖 Fig. 1.25).
- In another longitudinal observational study, BP levels were consistently lower in prisoners on Alcatraz than in prison guards.[2] Again, ordered, predictable lifestyles led by the prisoners, versus the more stressful occupations of the guards, was thought to explain the differences in BP.

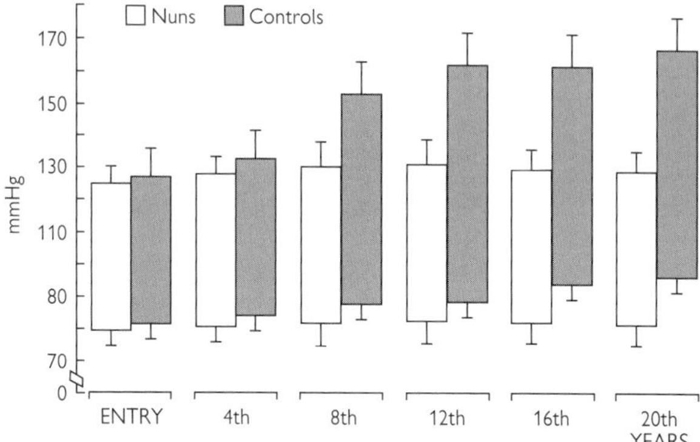

Fig. 1.25 Mean systolic and diastolic BPs in nuns in secluded orders versus controls. Adapted with permission from Timio M, *et al.* (1988). Age and blood pressure changes. A 20-year follow-up study in nuns in a secluded order. *Hypertension* **12**:457–61.

References

1. Timio M, *et al.* (1988). Age and blood pressure changes. A 20-year follow-up study in nuns in a secluded order. *Hypertension* **12**:457–61.
2. Alvarez WC and Stanley LL (1930). Blood pressure in 6000 prisoners and 400 guards. *Archives of Internal Medicine*, **46**:17–39.

Obesity

Population studies indicate a significant association between body weight or body mass index (BMI) and BP, even in normotensive individuals:

- The Framingham Heart Study demonstrated that SBP was ↑ by 6.5mmHg for every 10% ↑ in relative weight.[1]
- Studies examining the effects of weight loss on BP have observed that reductions in body weight of between 4.5–9kg led to reductions in BP of between 5–8mmHg (systolic) and 5–9mmHg (diastolic).[2]

The incidence of hypertension is ~50% in obese individuals (BMI >30kg/m^2) and obesity and hypertension frequently occur together in the metabolic syndrome. Recent data from the NHANES III survey suggest that BMI and weight gain over time are significant risk factors for the development of IDH.[3] Distribution of body fat may also be important, since upper body (central) fat is more closely associated with the development of hypertension than peripheral fat. Central obesity is also linked to insulin resistance, providing a link between obesity and glucose intolerance in the development of hypertension. Therefore, obesity is an important environmental factor associated with BP elevation and the growing prevalence of obesity in industrialized societies holds important implications for the future incidence and management of essential hypertension.

The mechanisms by which obesity contributes to the pathogenesis of hypertension are unclear but probably involve many factors (📖 Fig. 1.26). One such mechanism may be that the excessive dietary energy load in obese individuals stimulates the sympathetic nervous system, leading to an elevation in arterial pressure. Indeed, obese individuals exhibit selective activation of the renal sympathetic nerves compared with non-obese individuals, regardless of the level of BP. In contrast, cardiac sympathetic nervous system activity is ↑ in obese hypertensive individuals compared with obese normotensive individuals, suggesting that ↑ cardiac sympathetic outflow is an important feature of obesity-associated hypertension.

An intriguing question is whether hypertension might predispose individuals to the development of obesity later in life. Data from the Tecumseh study showed that elevated BPs preceded the ↑ in body fat in subjects with borderline hypertension (📖 Fig. 1.27).[4] A potential hypothesis explaining these observations is that enhanced sympathetic activation, which was also observed in the hypertensives at a young age, might lead to the development of insulin resistance and subsequent obesity later in life.

References

1. Kannel WB, Brand N, Skinner JJ *et al.* (1967). The relation of adiposity to blood pressure and development of hypertension. The Framingham Heart Study. *Ann Intern Med.* **67**:48–59.
2. Blumenthal JA, Sherwood A, Gullette EC *et al.* (2000). Exercise and weight loss reduce blood pressure in men and women with hypertension: effects on cardiovascular, metabolic and hemodynamic functioning. *Arch. Intern Med.* **160**:1947–58.
3. Franklin SS, Barboza MG, Pio JR, Wong ND (2006). Blood pressure categories, hypertensive sub-types and the metabolic syndrome. *J Hypertension*, **24**:2009–16.
4. Julius S, Jamerson K, Mejia A, *et al.* (1990). The association of borderline hypertension with target organ changes and higher coronary risk: TECUMSEH blood pressure study. *JAMA*, **264**:354–58.

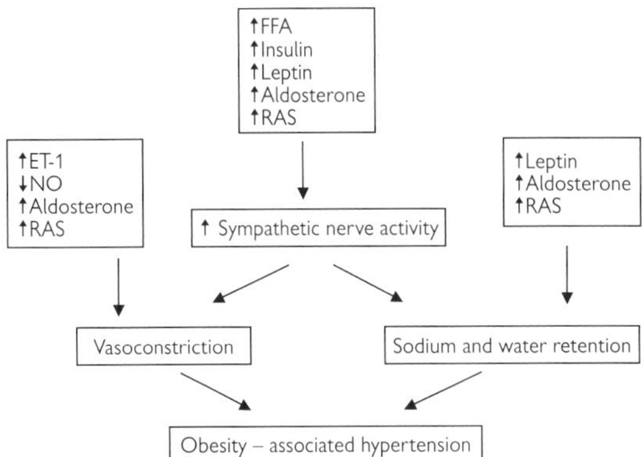

Fig. 1.26 Proposed mechanisms involved in obesity-associated hypertension. Data from Rahmouni K, *et al.* (2005). Obesity associated hypertension. *Hypertension* **45**:9–14.

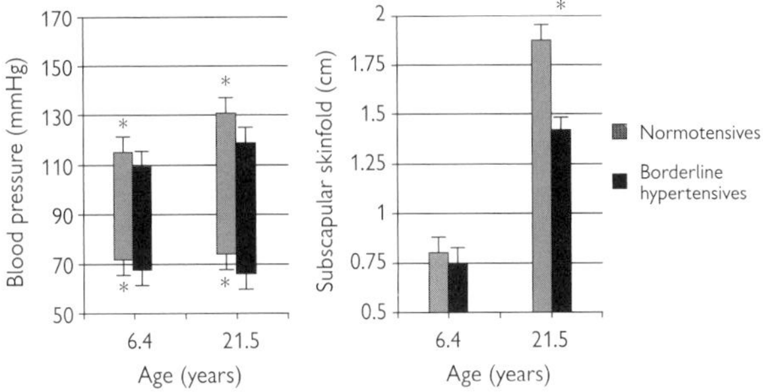

Fig. 1.27 Changes in BP and skinfold thickness over 15 years in normotensive and borderline hypertensive adults. Data from Julius S, *et al.* (1990). The association of borderline hypertension with target organ changes and higher coronary risk. Tecumseh Blood Pressure Study. *JAMA* **264**:354–8.

Experimental models of hypertension

Experimental models of hypertension allow detailed investigations into the causes of, and clinical signs associated with hypertension, as well as the effects of treatment to lower BP. The earliest experimental models of hypertension are largely attributed to the work of Goldblatt, who induced renal artery stenosis in dogs resulting in elevated BP (📖 Fig. 1.28):[1]

- One-kidney, one-clip model: one kidney is removed and a silver clip placed on the renal artery of the remaining kidney. The resulting occlusion causes a short-term rise in plasma renin activity, which then normalizes, and an ↑ plasma volume. Blockade of the RAAS does not reduce BP; however, diuresis and sodium depletion causes a return to the renin-dependent state, indicating a complex set of interactions between the RAAS and sodium retention by the kidney. This model represents bilateral renal artery stenosis in humans.
- Two-kidney, one-clip model: a silver clip is placed on one renal artery resulting in an ↑ renin secretion from the stenosed kidney and production of angiotensin II. Renin secretion from the intact kidney is either greatly reduced or absent. Administration of an angiotensin II antagonist normalizes BP in this model, indicating renin/angiotensin dependent hypertension, at least in its early phase.
- Two-kidney, two-clip model: this model exerts similar effects to the one-kidney, one-clip model except that the greater kidney mass in this model permits ↑ sodium excretion.
- Cellophane wrapping of the kidney: this model mimics renal capsular fibrosis, resulting in compression of the kidney and an ↑ in renal tissue pressure which ↓ renal blood flow and leads to the release of renin and angiotensin.

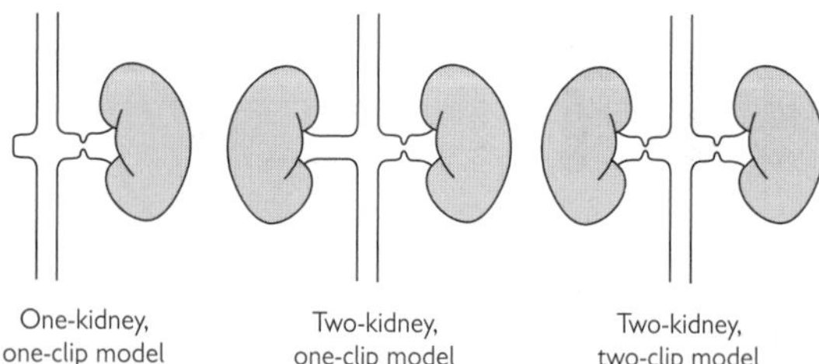

Fig. 1.28 Goldblatt's kidney–clip models of hypertension.

Genetic models

Genetic models allow the study of hypertension which develops spontaneously in an animal without any apparent cause, in order to mimic the situation in humans as closely as possible. This approach has the advantage that animals in which hypertension is a phenotype can be selectively bred, allowing the study of genes related to hypertension. A further advantage is that environmental influences on hypertension can be well controlled.

- Spontaneously hypertensive rats (SHR): a widely used model for studying hypertension. Developed by mating hypertensive 'progenitors' originally selected from Wistar rats from Kyoto in Japan (WK rats). WK rats are often used as normotensive controls in studies involving SHR. The SH stroke-prone rat is often used to study hypertension, stroke, and CVD.

- New Zealand genetically hypertensive rat: created by selective inbreeding for high BP and used as a model of hypertension and cardiac hypertrophy
- Dahl salt-sensitive and salt-resistant rats: selectively bred based on a tendency to either develop hypertension, or remain unaffected by alterations in dietary sodium intake. Salt-sensitive rats placed on a high sodium diet die within 8 weeks. When placed on a low salt diet, they die within 6 months.
- Milan hypertensive rat: descended from Wistar rats after selective breeding for hypertension. These rats provide a model of mild hypertension.
- Sabra hypertension-prone and hypertension-resistant rats: bred based on the propensity to develop hypertension or remain normotensive following 1 month on a high-salt diet.
- Lyon model of hypertension: 3 strains originally bred from Sprague–Dawley rats—hypertensive, normotensive, and a hypotensive model.
- Other strains related to hypertension: obesity–prone Sprague–Dawley rats, obese zucker rats, Wistar fatty rats.
- Other normotensive models: Brown Norway rats, Lewis rats, Fischer (F344) rats.

Reference

1. Goldblatt H, Lynch J, Hunzal RF, *et al.* (1934). Studies in experimental hypertension: I, The production of persistent elevation of systolic pressure by means of renal ischemia. *J Exp Med.* **59**:347–79.

Chapter 2

Essential hypertension

Prevalence and incidence

Hypertension is the commonest risk factor for CVD. It affects approximately 30% of the adult population globally and is thought to account for about 5% of adult deaths worldwide. However, it is much rarer in rural societies and practically non-existent in a few isolated communities, such as the natives of the Solomon Islands. In rural Indian men, hypertension is thought to occur in 3.4%[1].

The prevalence of essential hypertension rises dramatically with age in most Western communities, affecting 30% of men and women generally and rising up to >67% beyond the age of 75 years (📖 see Fig. 2.1). It also frequently occurs with other CV risk factors, especially diabetes mellitus, and this has formed the basis for the so-called metabolic syndrome.

There is some suggestion that the incidence of hypertension may have declined amongst students in Glasgow, UK between 1948–1968[2], which has led to a reduction in mortality from stroke. This may be due to effective population-based strategies to target CVD and may be important to translate across to undeveloped nations, who are likely to see a rise in CV mortality over the next few decades.

Hypertension is traditionally classified into primary (essential) or secondary (to an identifiable cause). However, this is an unsatisfactory classification because ~90% of hypertension is classified as essential, and it is very likely that subtypes of essential hypertension exist with different underlying mechanisms (📖 see Haemodynamics in hypertension, p.4). In some respects, essential hypertension is akin to a syndrome, i.e. there is no clear genetic, environmental, or other cause, and it is asymptomatic.

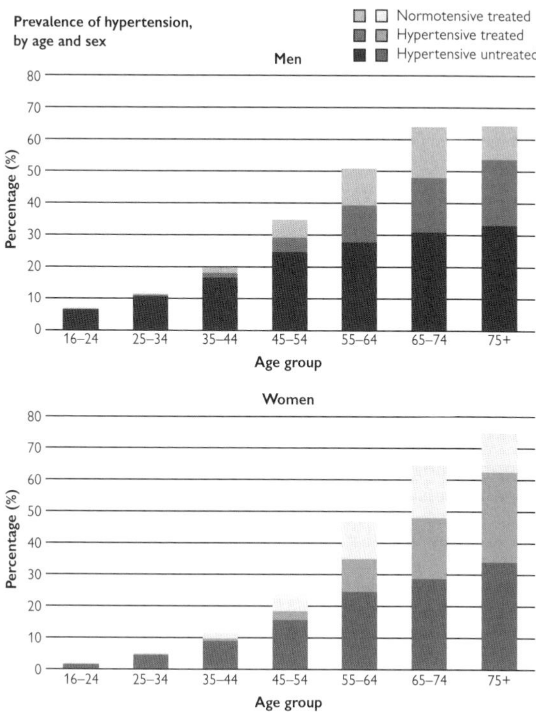

Fig. 2.1 Prevalence of hypertension by age and sex, Health Survey for England 2003. Reproduced under the terms of the Click-Use License.

References

1. Kearney PM, *et al.* (2004) Worldwide prevalence of hypertension. A systematic review. *J Hypertens* **22**:11–19.
2. McCarron P, *et al.* (2001) Change sin blood pressure among students attending Glasgow University between 1948 and 1968: analyses of cross sectional surveys. *BMJ* **322**:885–8.

Isolated systolic hypertension

Definition

ISH refers to the finding of a high SBP in the context of a normal or low DBP. The 'standard', but somewhat arbitrary, definition is a SBP ≥140mmHg, and DBP <90mmHg (BHS, WHO, JNC 7). ISH may be further divided into stage I SBP (140–159mmHg), and stage II SBP (≥160mmHg).

Prevalence

ISH is now the commonest form of hypertension in the UK and USA. The prevalence rises exponentially with age (Fig. 2.2), such that while only 7.4% of 40-year-olds are affected, ~30% of 60-year-olds and ~65% of those >80 years have ISH (≥140 & <90). Overall, ISH outnumbers other forms of hypertension by a factor of 2:1, but it is relatively less common in middle-aged people, and by far the most common form of hypertension in the over 60s (80% of all cases). The age-prevalence curve is shifted to the left in diabetics (📖 see Fig. 6.6), indicating that ISH tends to occur earlier in life. Interestingly there is also a second, much smaller, peak in the under 30s, where again it is the commonest form of hypertension.

Pathophysiology

Primarily the result of ↑ aortic stiffness; ↑ peripheral resistance does not seem to play a major role. Aortic stiffness rises exponentially with age (arteriosclerosis) in almost all societies mirroring the ↑ in the prevalence of ISH. The mechanisms responsible for arteriosclerosis are unclear but fatigue fracture of elastin, deposition of collagen, and medial calcification are probably all involved. It should be viewed as pathological—not simply part of normal ageing—because it is not observed in indigenous populations, and various risk factors for stiffening including female gender, diabetes, cigarette smoking, and previous 'borderline' or high normal BP have been identified. It is also important to recognize that ISH is not simply the 'burnt-out phase' of previous mixed SDH, since the majority of individuals do not have antecedent hypertension.

In young people, ISH can result from either a raised cardiac output, or aortic stiffening. Those primarily with an elevated cardiac output are likely to be in the early 'hyperdynamic' phase of essential hypertension. Previous long-term follow-up studies conducted in the 1970s suggest that over time, cardiac output falls back to normal, and peripheral resistance rises in such individuals. As a result, diastolic pressure rises and the syndrome of hypertension changes from predominant ISH to mixed SDH (📖 see Haemodynamics in hypertension, p.4). The mechanisms responsible for ↑ aortic stiffness in younger subjects are unclear, as is their long-term fate.

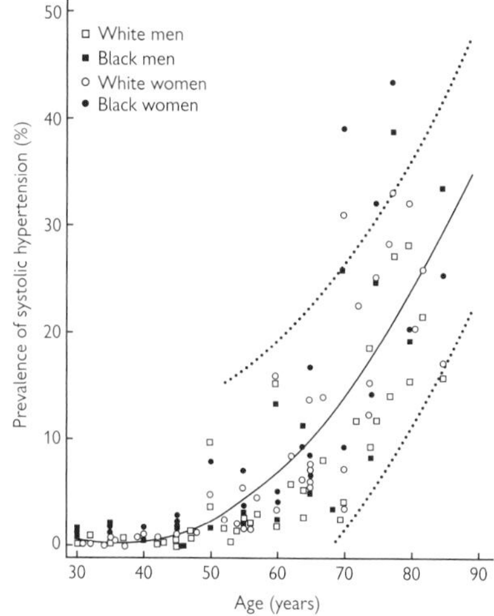

Fig. 2.2 Prevalence of ISH versus age in Europe (≥160 & <90 mmHg). Reproduced with permission from Staessen J, *et al.* (1990). Isolated systolic hypertension in the elderly. *J Hypertens* **8**:393–405.

Risks

Although ISH was previously considered benign, it is actually a major risk factor for stroke and CHD. A wealth of epidemiological data indicates that:

- There is a continuous relationship between SBP and risk of CV events at all ages.
- After the age of 55, there is an inverse relationship between DBP and risk, suggesting that individuals with ISH are at even greater risk compared to both normotensive subjects and those with SDH.
- ISH defined as SBP ≥160mmHg carries a 3-fold ↑ risk of stroke and a doubling in the risk of coronary heart disease (CHD). Those with stage I ISH are at intermediate risk.

Treatment

Benefits of BP reduction

Three randomized, placebo-controlled trials investigated the impact of BP lowering in patients with ISH (📖 Table 2.1). A meta-analysis of the 8 trials involving ISH found that overall active treatment reduced mortality by 13%, stroke by 30%, and CHD by 23%. Thus, treating older subjects with ISH compares favourably to treating younger subjects with mild hypertension. The number needed to treat (NNT) for stroke prevention of in older subjects is ~35 compared to a value of ~90 in younger subjects. Importantly, the incidence of side effects appears no more common in older subjects, including orthostatic hypotension. Limited data are available in subjects >80 years. However, a meta-analysis of ~1600 patients aged 80+ found significant reductions in the incidence of stroke, heart failure, but no effect of therapy on mortality. The Hypertension in the Very Elderly Trial (HYVET) recently confirmed the benefit of treating subjects >80 years of age with ISH.

Targets

No specific targets for ISH have been developed, and the majority of guidelines recommend similar targets for all essential hypertensives (140/85mmHg). However, SBP is more difficult to control than DBP (📖 Fig. 2.3). Consequently, subjects with ISH often end up on combination therapy, which may result in excessive DBP reduction and symptoms of breathlessness or angina. A retrospective analysis of the SHEP study[1] also suggested that a DBP <70mmHg on treatment is associated with an ↑ risk of events (📖 see Fig. 6.11, p.203). Practically, one should be cautious in producing excessive falls in DBP in older subjects with systolic hypertension, accepting that this may leave imperfect control of SBP.

Table 2.1 Summary of the 3 randomized, placebo-controlled trials in ISH

Trial	No. subjects	Treatment	↓ BP (mmHg)	↓ events
SHEP	4736	Chlorthalidone ± atenolol	11/3	Stroke 33% MI 33% CV death 20%* Death 13%*
SystEur	4695	Nitrendipine ± enalapril ± diuretic	10/4	Stroke 42% MI 30%* CV death 27%* Death 14%*
SystChina	1253	Nitrendipine ± captopril ± diuretic	9/3	Stroke 38% MI 1%* CV death 39% Death 39%

* = not significant. CV, cardiovascular; MI, myocardial infarction.

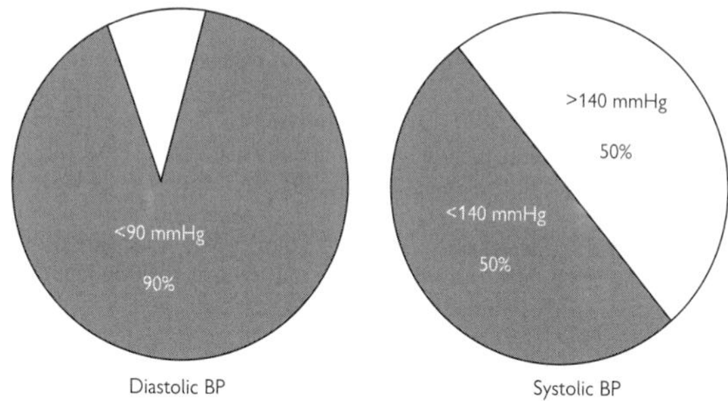

Fig. 2.3 No. of subjects achieving DBP<90 mmHg or SBP <140 mmHg. Data from Mancia G and Grassi G. (2002). Systolic and diastolic blood pressure control in antihypertensive drug trials. *J Hypertens* **20**:1461–4.

Reference

1. Shorr RI and Somes GW (2000). Can diastolic blood pressure be excessively lowered in the treatment of isolated systolic hypertension? *J Clini Hyper* **2**:134–7.

Choice of drug

Placebo-controlled evidence exists for the use of thiazide diuretics (SHEP) and long-acting calcium blockers (SystEur/China) in ISH. However, several other studies have included a large proportion of ISH subjects and used other therapies first-line, including β-blockers, ACEI, and ARAs. No study has addressed directly the question of drug superiority in ISH subjects. STOP-2 included a large proportion of ISH subjects and found no difference between thiazides/β-blockers, ACEIs, and calcium blockers. A subgroup analysis of ALLHAT found the same, but did not include β-blockers. Several recent studies, the MRC Elderly Study, and meta-analyses indicate that β-blockers may be less effective than other drugs. Therefore, on balance, it seems that with the exception of β-blockers the 3 main classes of drugs are equally effective. Three randomized studies also suggest that nitrates may be of benefit in subjects with ISH although they have not been subject to long-term trials. α-blockers may precipitate orthostatic hypotension—especially in those with very wide pulse pressure and stiff arteries—and should be used with caution. A schema for the logical combination of drugs is shown in 📖 Fig. 2.4.

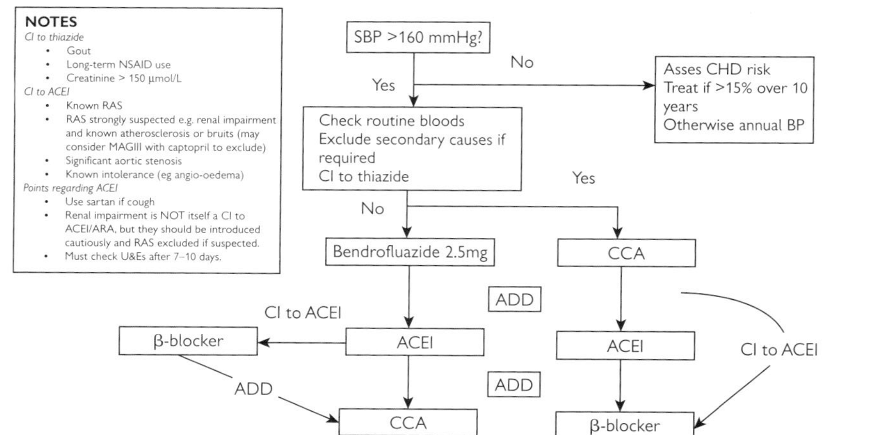
Treatment Guideline for ISH
(SBP>140 AND DBP<90mmHg)
NOTES
CI to thiazide
• Gout
• Long-term NSAID use
• Creatinine > 150 μmol/L
CI to ACEI
• Known RAS
• RAS strongly suspected e.g. renal impairment and known atherosclerosis or bruits (may consider MAGIII with captopril to exclude)
• Significant aortic stenosis
• Known intolerance (eg angio-oedema)
Points regarding ACEI
• Use sartan if cough
• Renal impairment is NOT itself a CI to ACEI/ARA, but they should be introduced cautiously and RAS excluded if suspected.
• Must check U&Es after 7–10 days.
SBP >160 mmHg?
No
Yes
Asses CHD risk
Treat if >15% over 10 years
Otherwise annual BP
Check routine blood
Exclude secondary causes if required
CI to thiazide
Yes
No
Bendrofluazide 2.5mg
CCA
ADD
CI to ACEI
β-blocker
ACEI
ACEI
CI to ACEI
ADD
ADD
CCA
β-blocker

Fig. 2.4 Suggested treatment algorithm for ISH. ACEI, angiotension-converting enzyme inhibitor; CI, contraindications; NSAID, non-steroidal anti-inflammatory drug. RAS, renal artery stenosis.

Systolic/diastolic hypertension

Definition

Mixed SDH refers to an elevation of systolic and diastolic BP. This is the classical form of hypertension and is often viewed as 'established' or fixed hypertension. SDH can be further classified into two or three stages (📖 Table 2.2), depending on the definition used.

Table 2.2 Categorization of SDH

Stage 1:	SBP 140–159mmHg & DBP 90–99mmHg BHS/JNC7
Stage 2:	SBP ≥160mmHg & DBP ≥100mmHg BHS/JNC7
Stage 3:	SBP ≥180mmHg & DBP ≥110mmHg BHS

Prevalence

SDH is the most prevalent form of hypertension in middle-aged individuals, with ~18% of 40-year-olds affected. Although the prevalence ↑ to ~30% in 60-year-olds, ISH is by far the most common form of essential hypertension in the older population. A modest proportion of patients (~20%) may transform from SDH into ISH in later life. Similarly, IDH and ISH predominate in the under 30s and often change into SDH later.

Pathophysiology

Unlike ISH, SDH is associated with a marked ↑ in PVR. In most individuals, this is thought to evolve from an early elevation in cardiac output, causing a rise in BP—a marked feature of patients with 'early' or 'borderline' hypertension. Cardiac output normalizes over time, giving way to a more sustained rise in PVR, which most likely develops in response to the continuous exposure to elevated BP.

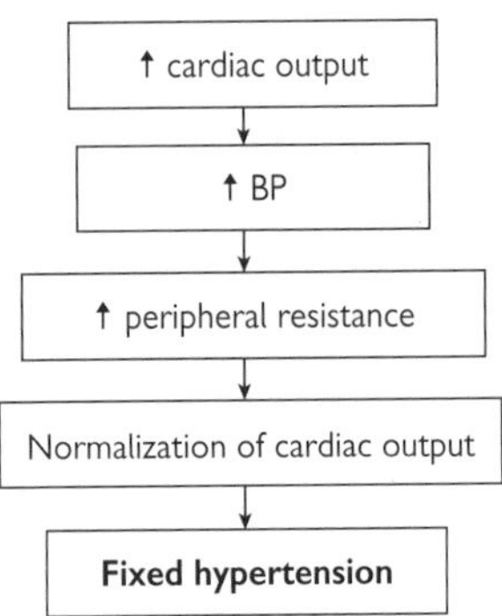

Fig. 2.5 Haemodynamic abnormalities leading to SDH.

Isolated diastolic hypertension

Definition

IDH refers to an elevated DBP in the presence of a normal SBP. Although this form of hypertension is frequently overlooked in general guidelines for the classification of hypertension, in practice, IDH is defined as a SBP of <140mmHg and a DBP ≥90mmHg.

Prevalence

When considered as a separate sub-type of hypertension, IDH is the most common form of diastolic hypertension in individuals <40 years. Moreover, data from NHANES III suggest that in younger individuals (<50 years) IDH accounts for ~40% of all hypertension (📖 see Fig. 1.2, p.5).

Pathophysiology

IDH is thought to evolve primarily from normal or high-normal BP. Follow-up studies suggest that individuals with IDH later develop mixed SDH. As in mixed hypertension, an ↑ PVR is thought to be an important haemodynamic feature of IDH. Interestingly, IDH is strongly associated with ↑ BMI and weight gain over time, suggesting shared links with obesity and the metabolic syndrome. Indeed, data from the NHANES III survey in the USA demonstrate a strong association between IDH and risk factors for the metabolic syndrome in young adult men and women. These findings contrast with previous suggestions that IDH is a benign condition, devoid of CV risk.

History

The clinical history may provide clues as to the aetiology of hypertension and provide a guide to subsequent management.

Background

It is important to establish when the hypertension was first noted, whether the readings were consistently elevated or not, and the relationship to other extraneous factors e.g. stress, anxiety, etc.

General

In the vast majority, hypertension is generally asymptomatic. Associated symptoms often suggest 2° hypertension, e.g. sweating, palpitations, labile BP, feelings of impending doom may suggest a phaeochromocytoma (📖 see Box 2.1). A paradoxical ↑ in BP on β-blockade also suggests a phaeochromocytoma due to unopposed α-mediated vasoconstriction.

Box 2.1 Symptoms of phaeochromocytoma

- Headache.
- Sweating attacks accompanied by pallor.
- Palpitations.
- Feelings of anxiety.
- Chest pain.
- Abdominal pain.
- Nausea.
- Vomiting.
- Weight loss.
- Breathlessness.
- Blurred vision.
- Dizziness.
- Faints.
- Seizures.

On the other hand, tremor, palpitations, sweating, weight loss, etc. may suggest thyrotoxicosis. A worsening renal function on ACEIs or angiotensin receptor antagonists (ARAs) may point to renovascular disease or RAS. Renovascular hypertension should also be considered in those presenting either aged >60 years or <30 years associated with a renal bruit, drug-resistant hypertension or recurrent pulmonary oedema. Headaches, non-specific abdominal pains and haematospermia are sometimes seen in cases of accelerated phase hypertension.

Risk factors

Lifestyle issues such as a poor diet (e.g. fatty foods, processed diets) and exercise should be interrogated. Excess salt intake as well as alcohol may contribute to hypertension as does liquorice! A sedentary lifestyle, smoking, and obesity ↑ the risks for the development of CVD—so these should be considered as important adjuncts to target in the management of the hypertensive patient.

Past medical history

A previous history of CV event (e.g. previous angina, MI, stroke, TIA, or peripheral vascular disease) ↑ the risk of future events, especially if the patient's hypertension remains uncontrolled and alters the target pressure to be achieved. Other concomitant features which ↑ CV risk—including racial origins, hypercholesterolaemia, renal failure, and diabetes mellitus—should also be elucidated. A past medical history of pre-eclampsia or pregnancy-induced hypertension may be useful in determining the aetiology of hypertension.

Drug history

A previous or current drug history is vital, as well as a record of the patient's side effects to particular therapies or class of therapies. Compliance is a major factor in BP control, so this should be assessed adequately, perhaps with a collateral history. It may be important to emphasize the relative importance of therapy (in terms of risk reduction) versus some, possibly trivial, side effects—although it remains important to listen to the patient and come to an understanding of their issues pertaining to drug therapy. Other concomitant drugs, e.g. oral contraceptives, may exacerbate hypertension, so it may be prudent to have a trial of withdrawing this to see if it is indeed pill-induced hypertension (📖 see also Oral contraceptive pill, p.165). Other drugs include NSAIDs, steroids, and so on (📖 see drugs discussed in Chapter 4, pp.165–168). Resistant hypertension is defined as a failure to achieve BP targets despite 3 or more antihypertensive agents.

Family history

This may point to an underlying genetic cause although this is very rare.

Examination

A thorough physical examination is vital at the initial consultation as it may reveal some important clues in diagnosing 2° causes and underlying risk factors. It also picks up target organ damage which lowers the target BP to be achieved.

General

- Height, weight, and BMI (weight ÷ height^2 in kg/m^2).
- Presence of corneal arcus—hypercholesterolaemia in a young patient (🕮 see Colour plate 1).
- Xanthomata and xanthelasma (🕮 see Colour plate 2 and 3).
- Nicotine staining—smoking.
- Cushingoid facies, a buffalo hump—Cushing's syndrome.
- Lid lag, lid retraction, tremor with atrial fibrillation (AF)—thyrotoxicosis.

Cardiorespiratory

- Pulse for rate, rhythm (?AF), pulse delays (radiofemoral), and check for a full complement of pulses—a delayed pulse may indicate a coarctation of the aorta.
- BP should be checked in both arms in the seated position and when standing—after 2–3min for any significant postural drop.
- Jugular venous pulse and signs of peripheral oedema—to assess fluid status.
- Ventricular failure or valvular dysfunction which may represent a previous myocardial event. Type A aortic dissection—aortic regurgitation.
- Pulmonary oedema or wheeze which may restrain potential β-blockade therapy.

Abdominal

- Renal bruits—renovascular disease or fibromuscular dysplasia.
- Expansile and pulsatile mass may suggest an abdominal aortic aneurysm.
- Ballotable kidneys—polycystic kidney disease or hypernephroma.

Neurological

- Full neurological examination—previous stroke or in an emergency with an acute aortic dissection.
- Mental state examination—underlying dementia, e.g. from multi-infarct dementia.

Fundoscopy

- Hypertensive retinopathy reflects the changes seen due to systemic hypertension and is therefore usually bilateral. Graded according to the Keith–Wagener–Barker classification system in 1939 but now superseded by a newer system as detailed in 🕮 Table 2.3.
- Diabetic retinopathy—may suggest underlying previous undiagnosed diabetes mellitus.

Table 2.3 Classification of hypertensive retinopathy

Grade of retinopathy	Changes seen
I	Silver wiring
II	Grade I + arteriovenous nipping
III	Grade II + cotton wool spots, retinal oedema, haemorrhages
IV	Grade III + optic disc swelling

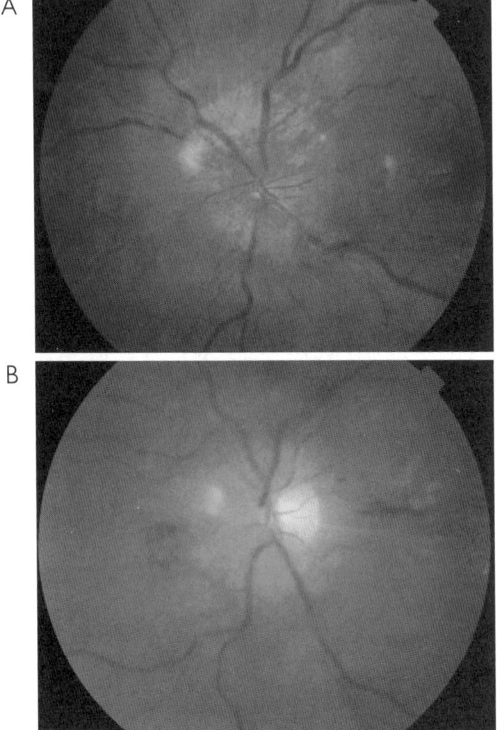

Fig. 2.6 Grade IV hypertensive retinopathy with optic disc swelling, haemorrhages, soft exudates, and retinal oedema (📖 see also Colour plates 4–6).

Blood pressure measurement

This is vital to reaching the correct diagnosis. Only validated machines should be used. A list of these can be obtained from the BHS website.[1] See also the BHS guidelines on the correct technique for measurement.[2]

Anaeroid sphygmomanometers should be avoided. Other automated machines (e.g. oscillometric) should be validated—although it is worthwhile remembering that some of these machines may not be able to measure BP accurately in AF or at extreme BP.

The BP cuff should be an appropriate size for the patient to cover 80% of the upper arm. It may be worthwhile to measure the circumference of the patient's upper arm halfway up to ensure the appropriate-sized cuff is being used. Otherwise BP may be over- or underestimated. Larger cuffs are required for obese subjects and smaller ones in paediatrics.

The patient should be rested for at least 5–10min in the seated position in a quiet room. They should not be talking during the measurements nor crossing their legs. Their arm should be at the same level as their heart and be supported.

Manual sphygmomanometry

- Ensure there is no parallax between the observer and the machine.
- Inflate the cuff to suprasystolic (to obliterate the radial pulse) to give an idea of the SBP. Then deflate and re-inflate to 30mmHg above this estimated figure and deflate slowly (2–3mmHg/sec).
- Korotkoff I indicating SBP is when the first sound is heard.
- The disappearance of sounds (Korotkoff V) is DBP (although in some people, this does not ever disappear, in which case, muffling of the sounds at Korotkoff IV is taken as the DBP).
- Record BP to the nearest 2mmHg.

References

1. Validated blood pressure monitors list from the BHS website: http://www.bhsoc.org/blood_pressure_list.stm
2. BHS guidelines: http://www.bhsoc.org/how_to_measure_blood_pressure.stm

Assessing end-organ damage

End-organ damage or target organ damage (TOD) essentially implies the end result of sustained hypertension resulting in a variety of pathophysiological changes in various organs of the body. The continued shear stress results in endothelial dysfunction, ↑ risk of thrombogenesis, accelerated atherosclerosis, and finally culminating in a CV event.

At a macroscopic level, the larger arteries stiffen and display reduced compliance. The more peripheral arteries have reduced lumen size and result in a continuing cycle of worsening hypertension by ↑ systemic peripheral resistance. This ↑ the afterload and left ventricular work ↑—leading to LVH. The ↑ prothrombotic state is evidenced by a variety of factors including von Willebrand factor, fibrinogen, and so on. This may result in occlusive events, e.g. TIAs or strokes.

Atherosclerosis may present in terms of peripheral vascular disease, strokes, MI or angina, renal disease (📖 see also Colour plate 15), or retinal occlusion.

Assessment of TOD should be directed according to the history and examination and evidence may be obtained as per Box 2.2.

Box 2.2 Assessing end-organ damage

CV

Electrocardiogram (ECG).
Echocardiography.
Chest X-ray (CXR).
Coronary angiography.
Cardiac magnetic resonance imaging (MRI).

Renal

Dipstick urinalysis and microscopy.
Microalbuminuria.
Serum creatinine and estimated glomerular filtration rate (eGFR).
Ultrasound scan (USS)—renal.

Neurology

USS—carotids.
Computed tomography (CT)/MRI—brain.

Ophthalmology

Fundoscopy.
Visual field tests (📖 Fig 2.7).
Fluorescein angiography.

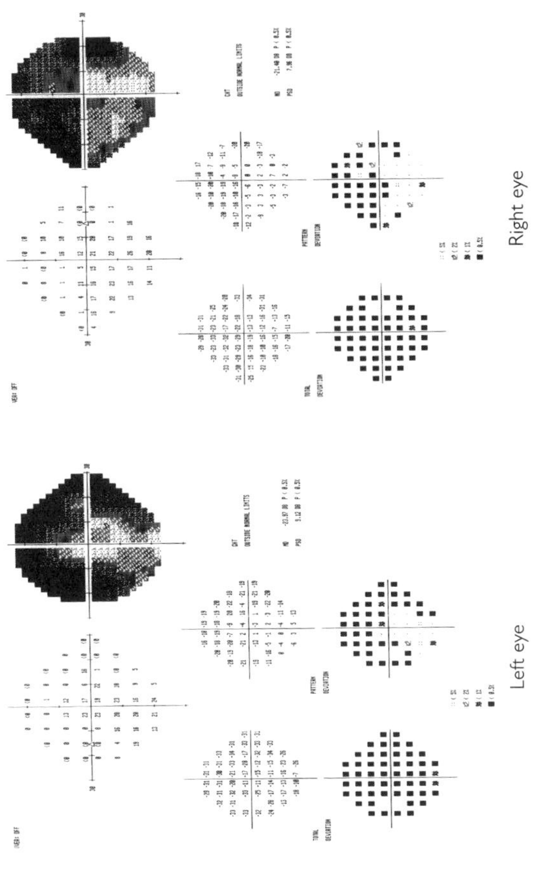

Fig. 2.7 Visual field testing reveals bilateral lower visual field defects in a patient with papilloedema.

Investigations in hypertension

Investigations should be guided by history and examination and to search for TOD. They can be grouped into standard screening tests to assess other CV risk factors and those specific to screen for common 2° causes. Specific investigations are generally performed to exclude 2° causes.

General (for all patients)

- Urea and electrolytes (U&Es).
- Glucose.
- Liver function tests (LFTs).
- Thyroid function tests (TFTs).
- Comprehensive lipid profile.
- Full blood count (FBC).
- Erythrocyte sedimentation rate (ESR).
- Urinalysis (protein, blood, glucose).
- 12-lead ECG.
- CXR only if suspecting aortic coarctation or dissection.

Specific

Blood

- Bicarbonate.
- Renin and aldosterone.
- Autoimmune profile:
    - Anti-neutrophilic cytoplasmic antibodies (ANCAs).
    - Antinuclear antibodies (ANAs).
    - Double-stranded (ds)-DNA.
    - Anti-glomerular basement membrane (GBM).
    - Immunoglobulin (Ig) electrophoresis.
- Plasma catecholamines.
- Parathyroid hormone (PTH) and repeat calcium if initial corrected calcium is abnormal.

Urine

- 24-h urine vanillylmandelic acid (VMA) or metanephrines.
- 24-h urine hydroxyindoleacetic acid (HIAA).
- 24-h urine Na^+, K^+, and creatinine clearance.
- 24-h urine free cortisol.

CV risk assessment

- Echocardiography.
- 24-h BP monitor.
- Exercise tolerance test.

Vascular hypertension

- CT angiography of subclavian vessels.

Endocrine hypertension

- Dexamethasone suppression test.
- CT/MRI adrenals.
- Adrenal vein sampling.

Suppression tests for phaeochromocytoma
- Clonidine or pentolinium suppression test.
- Dexamethasone suppression test.

Other tests for phaeochromocytoma
- MIBG scan.
- 3,4-dihydroxy-6-fluoro-DL-phenylananine (F-DOPA)/F-18 fluorodeoxy-glucose (FDG)-positron emission tomography (PET)-CT scans.

Renovascular/renally driven hypertension
- USS—abdomen.
- Mercapto-acetyltriglycine (MAG-3) renogram.
- Renal vein sampling.
- CT angiography of renal vessels.
- MR angiogram.
- Renal vein sampling.
- Dimercaptosuccinic acid (DMSA) scan.

Basic biochemistry

U&Es

Routine biochemistry for U&Es and creatinine is useful prior to therapy, to monitor the effects of therapy and to rule out 2° causes.

A ↓ K^+ with or without a ↑ Na^+ and ↑ HCO_3^- in the context of a patient not on diuretic therapy must alert the clinician to the possibility of an adrenal cause of hypertension or 2° hyperaldosteronism (📖 Box 2.3).

Box 2.3 Basic biochemistry and clues to 2° hypertension

↓ *K^+*
- 1° and 2° hyperaldosteronism.
- Cushing's syndrome.
- Liddle's syndrome.
- RAS/disease.

↑ *K^+*
- Exclude artefacts (e.g. delayed analyses).
- Unmasked by ACEI/ARA—RAS/disease.
- Renal failure.
- Immunosuppression.
- Thrombocythaemia.

↓ *Na^+*
- Diuretics.
- Syndrome of inappropriate antidiuretic hormone (SIADH) secretion.
- Intracranial pathology.
- Hypothyroidism.
- Hyperparathyroidism.

↑ *Na^+*
- Dehydration.
- 1° and 2° hyperaldosteronism.

↑ *creatinine*
- After commencement or dose escalation of ACEI or ARA should prompt investigation of RAS as an underlying cause.
- At the time of presentation with malignant hypertension indicates a poorer prognosis especially if the serum creatinine ≥300mmol/mL (📖 Fig. 2.8).

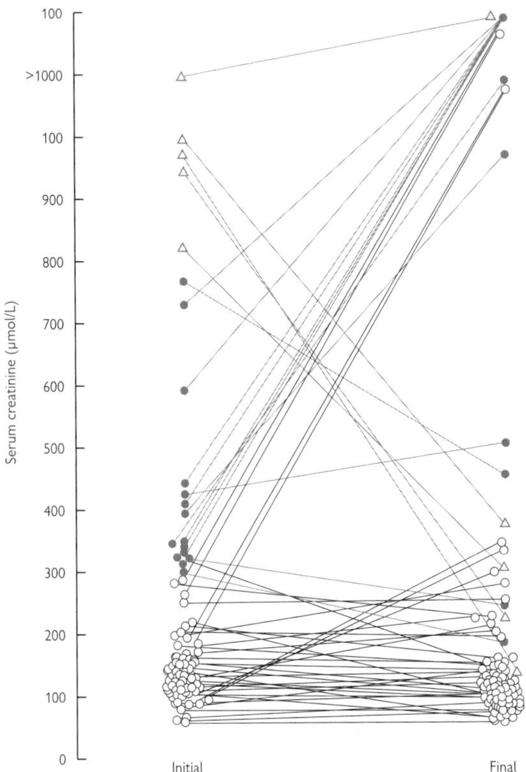

Fig. 2.8 Progression to end-stage renal failure in accelerated phase hypertension is dependent on presenting creatinine. ○ indicate patients whose serum creatinine was <300mmol/L; △ are those who presented with malignant hypertension and acute oliguric renal failure; and ● represent those presenting with chronic renal failure not requiring immediate dialysis. Adapted from Isles CG (1988). Malignant hypertension. In Catto GRD (ed.) *Management of Renal Hypertension. New Clinical Applications: Nephrology*. Lancaster: MTP Press, pp. 41–78, with kind permission of Springer Science and Business Media.

Renin and aldosterone

The availability of plasma renin activity assays and plasma aldosterone levels has revolutionized the modern management of hypertension. However, these should be interpreted with caution in the context of a patient already on drug therapy, particularly β-blockade.

β-blockers ↓ renin secretion at the juxtaglomerular apparatus so a ↓ renin on β-blockade is hardly surprising. However, a ↑ renin in this setting must raise the possibility of either non-compliance or renin-driven hypertension, e.g. RAS or nephrogenic causes including, very rarely, a reninoma. Conversely, most other drug therapies ↑ renin levels, so a ↓ renin in this setting may point to an adrenal cause of hypertension.

Similarly, an ↑ aldosterone must be interpreted in the context of the corresponding renin level. 2° hyperaldosteronism is strikingly common especially in the context of accelerated phase hypertension. A ↓ renin and ↑ aldosterone in a patient off β-blockade points to hyperaldosteronism as a cause for hypertension and further investigation should be undertaken to elucidate the cause. Beware that calcium-channel antagonists (CCAs) may mask the diagnosis with an apparently normal plasma aldosterone.[1]

The ratio of plasma aldosterone to renin (ARR) has been suggested as a useful screening tool for hyperaldosteronism. Apart from various factors such as posture and serum K^+ levels, antihypertensive therapies may cause false positive or false negative results. It may sometimes be necessary to alter therapies prior to making any assumptions on ARR *per se*.

Other biochemistry

It is also perhaps important to measure a patient's glucose level to rule out diabetes as a co-existing risk factor, especially in risk stratification. Thyroid and parathyroid function is also an easy, yet clinically important and treatable cause of hypertension that must not be forgotten, as is the case with ↑ Ca^{2+} and its underlying causes.

Reference

1. Brown MJ, *et al.* (1999). Calcium channel blockade can mask the diagnosis of Conn's syndrome. *Postgrad Med J* **75**:235–6.

Dipstick urinalysis

Dipstick urinalysis is a simple bedside test which can reveal underlying frank proteinuria as well as an active urinary sediment which may point to a renal cause for hypertension. It is also an important risk factor for subsequent renal failure, CVD, and is also correlated with overall mortality in hypertensive patients.

Microalbuminuria and proteinuria

As with diabetic patients, microalbuminuria (defined as a urinary albumin excretion of 20–200mg/L) is considered to be a sensitive marker of early, non-specific kidney damage. A spot urine albumin (μg)/creatinine (mg) ratio (ACR) is a convenient method of measuring microalbuminuria.

Microalbuminuria is:

- more closely related to ambulatory BP than clinic pressure.
- correlates with left ventricular mass and retinopathy.
- reverses with effective antihypertensive therapies suggesting that microalbuminuria (like LVH) may be a useful measure of end-organ damage and CV risk in hypertensive patients.

However, data from large trials are lacking and at present the true predictive value of microalbuminuria is uncertain. Nevertheless, the presence of microalbuminuria in a hypertensive patient should prompt a more detailed search for evidence of other end-organ damage.

A dipstick proteinuria of 3+ or more has a sensitivity of 96% and specificity of 87% of predicting a protein:creatinine ratio of ≥1—which is as good a surrogate of proteinuria as a 24-h urine collection.[1]

Haematuria

Microscopic haematuria is also a marker of hypertensive renal damage, although it is less closely related to clinical outcome than proteinuria. Hyaline arteriosclerosis, focal glomerular obsolescence, and thickening of GBMs are some of the nephrogenic changes that may result in dipstick haematuria. This can be associated with ↓ glomerular filtration, red blood cell casts, and persistent microscopic haematuria. Haematuria is also associated with some forms of renal parenchymal disease, and may, therefore, suggest an underlying cause for hypertension.

Glycosuria

Dipstick glycosuria needs little further mention apart from the obvious need to check fasting sugar levels and glycosylated haemoglobin to measure the long-term glycaemic control of an individual patient.

Laboratory testing for urinary albumin excretion and urine albumin: creatinine ratios are mandatory annually in all diabetic and renal patients.

Reference

1. Agarwal R, *et al.* (2002). Dipstick proteinuria: can it guide hypertension management? *Am J Kid Dis* **39**:1190–9.

Electrocardiography

A 12-lead ECG should be performed in all patients. It is a rough-and-ready screen for LVH and may also indicate previous myocardial damage, heart block, or dysrhythmias.

LVH is present in longstanding hypertension. In slim patients, the presence of LVH is often a false-positive finding when investigated further. Whilst ECGs are easy to perform, they are not as sensitive as cardiac MRI or modern echocardiography in picking up LVH (📖 Table 2.4).

LVH is the physiological result of myocardial stress pumping against an ↑ afterload in the form of PVR. In hypertension, this usually consists of concentric hypertrophy of the left ventricular wall and septum although other forms such as eccentric or asymmetric hypertrophy may occur.

LVH remains an important endpoint when considering treatment as it is linked to mortality outcomes in hypertension.[1] It is one of the major end-organ damage criteria in determining need for therapy in hypertension. Hence, its diagnosis requires careful consideration and evaluation.

Criteria

A variety of criteria have been developed to classify LVH (📖 see Box 2.4). The easiest and most readily used one is the Sokolow–Lyon index. A strain pattern indicated by ST depression and T-wave inversion in V4–6 is strongly supportive of LVH and may represent an ischaemic bulky left ventricle (📖 see Box 2.5). Left-axis deviation may also be present (📖 Fig. 2.9).

Metabolic disturbances may also be evident on the ECG. This can provide clues to the underlying diagnosis or side effects of therapy (📖 see Box 2.6).

Table 2.4 Sensitivity and specificity of ECG versus other modalities for LVH*

	ECG	M-mode	2-D Echo	3-D Echo	Cardiac MRI
Cost	low	moderate	moderate	moderate	high
Sensitivity	low	moderate	high	high	high
Specificity	high	high	high	high	high
Availability	high	high	high	low	low
Complexity	low	low	moderate	moderate	moderate

*Adapted with permission from Alfakih K, *et al.* (2006). The assessment of left ventricular hypertrophy in hypertension. *Hypertension* **24**:1223–30, Lippincott, Williams and Wilkins.

Box 2.4 LVH classification systems

Sokolow–Lyon[2]
S V1 + R V5 or V6 >35mm.

Cornell criteria[3]
S V3 + R aVL >28mm in men.
S V3 + R aVL >20mm in women.

Framingham criteria[4]
R aVL>11mm, R V4–6 >25mm.
S V1–3 >25 mm; S V1 or V2 + R V5 or V6 >35mm; R I + S III >25mm.

Box 2.5 Other causes of LVH and strain pattern

- Hypertrophic obstructive cardiomyopathy (HOCM).
- Aortic stenosis.
- True posterior infarction.
- Wolff–Parkinson–White Type A.

Box 2.6 ECG manifestations of metabolic abnormalities

- ↓ K^+: U waves (📖 Fig 2.10)—this may be a clue to underlying hyperaldosteronism. ST segment depression, QRS prolongation may also be present. Arrhythmias, e.g. ventricular ectopics, atrial tachycardia, heart block, ventricular tachycardia (VT), and ventricular fibrillation (VF) may also occur. ↓ Mg^{2+}may show similar features.
- ↑ K^+: tall, pointed T waves which are narrow, ↓ P-wave amplitude, ST segment changes, 1st-degree heart block, bundle branch blocks, VT, VF, asystole! ↑ Mg^{2+} may show similar features.
- ↑ Ca^{2+}: short QT.
- ↓ Ca^{2+}: long QT.

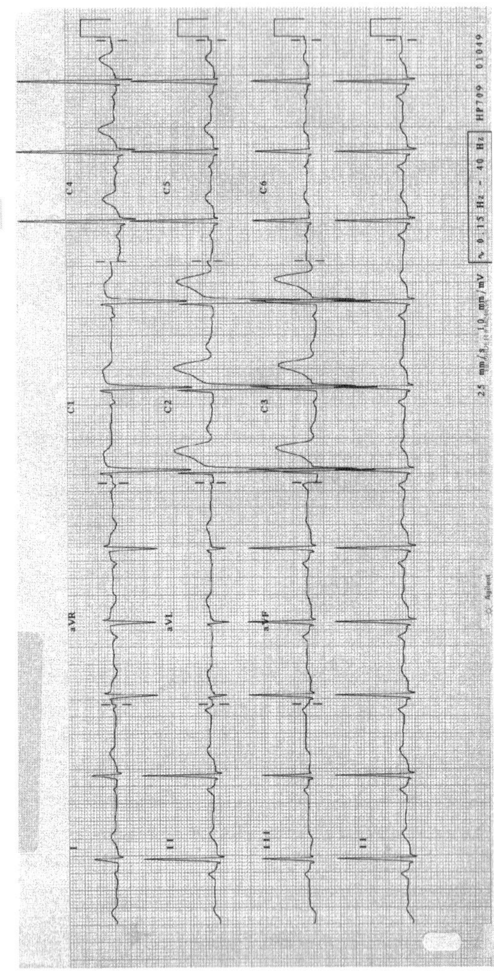

Fig. 2.9 LVH on voltage criteria.

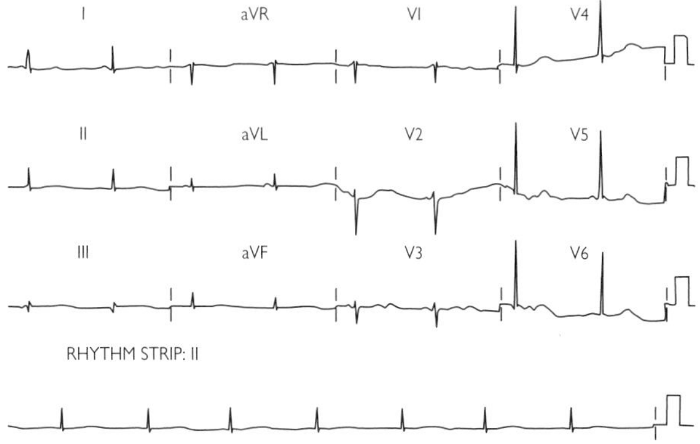

Fig. 2.10 U waves on 12-lead ECG indicating possible ↓ K^+.

References

1. Kannel WB, *et al.* (1970). Electrocardiographic left ventricular hypertrophy and risk of coronary heart disease. The Framingham Study. *Ann Intern Med* **72**:813–22.
2. Sokolow M and Lyon T (1949). The ventricular complex in left ventricular hypertrophy as obtained by unipolar precordial and limb leads. *Am Heart J* **37**:161–86.
3. Casale PN, *et al.* (1987). Improved sex-specific criteria of left ventricular hypertrophy for clinical and computer interpretation of electrocardiograms: validation with autopsy findings. *Circulation* **75**:565–72.
4. Levy D, *et al.* (1990). Determinants of sensitivity and specificity of electrocardiographic criteria for left ventricular hypertrophy. *Circulation* **81**:815–20.

Home blood pressure

Home monitoring is generally reliable if patients correctly use a well maintained, validated automated sphygmomanometer for measuring BP at the brachial artery (i.e. not radial etc.). A list of these can be obtained from the BHS website.[1]

Home monitoring can shorten the time taken for diagnosis and to achieve target pressure once therapy has been initiated. It is less validated for prognosis than ambulatory BP monitoring (ABPM) and the usual difference between home and clinic readings is unclear. Thresholds should be adjusted accordingly (📖 see THOP Trial[2]). Generally, this is accepted as being 10/5mmHg lower than clinic pressure measurements (as with ABPMs)—so a clinic target of 140/90mmHg is equivalent to a home target of 130/85mmHg.

Home BPs may ultimately gain ground over ABPMs due to ease of use, cheaper cost, and the convenience both for clinical trial purposes and clinical use. The American Society of Hypertension has recently issued a position statement on home blood pressure which may have implications for future practice.[3]

References

1. Automatic digital blood pressure devices for clinical use and also suitable for home/self assessment. Available at the BHS website: http://www.bhsoc.org/bp_monitors/automatic.stm
2. Staessen JA, *et al.* (2004). Antihypertensive treatment based on blood pressure measurement at home or in the physician's office: a randomized controlled trial. *JAMA* **291**:955–64.
3. Pickering TG, *et al.* (2008). ASH Positron Paper. Home and ambulatory blood pressure monitoring, when and how to use self (home) and ambulatory blood pressure monitoring. *J Clin Hypertens.* **10**(11):850–5.

24-hour ambulatory blood pressure monitoring

24-h ABPM is being used more widely and there are now several validated devices available (for a comprehensive list of these, please refer to the BHS website[1]). However, ABPM is not necessary for either diagnosis or management in the majority of hypertensive patients. The benefits of antihypertensive therapy in reducing CV risk have been almost exclusively established using seated clinic BP recordings.

Potential advantages

ABPMs offer the chance of a quicker patient diagnosis by accumulating multiple recordings of BP over a short time period and may provide faster monitoring of responses to changes in treatment. They are also a practical way of excluding white coat hypertension (📖 see Definitions).The inconvenience they pose comes partly from the frequency of recommended intervals (every 30min!)—which cannot be relaxing or comfortable, especially for patients who find the inflating cuffs painful or who have high pressure.

Whilst ABPM values may be closely associated with surrogate measures such as LVH and carotid intima-media thickness, there are insufficient outcome data concerning ABPM. However, those that are available suggest superiority, especially of nocturnal BP, over clinic BP.

Practical points

- These are invariably lower than clinic BP and thus an individual with a daytime ABPM average of 150/100mmHg is probably at more risk than a subject with the same clinic pressure.
- The accepted difference is that daytime ABPMs are ~10/5–12/7mmHg lower than clinic BP.
- Daytime average ABPM values are the most important comparator to clinic BP for management decisions. A 'normal' daytime average ABPM is defined as <135/85mmHg, but optimal values are <130/80mmHg (lower in diabetics).
- A normal dip is thought to be around 10% of daytime readings. Nighttime readings may be a stronger predictor than clinic, daytime, or average ABPMs (📖 Fig. 2.12). However, note the reversal of pattern in shift workers is usual. A lack of dipping may indicate poor sleep patterns due to obstructive sleep apnoea, prostatism, etc.

Definitions

- *White coat hypertension*: the clinic BP is elevated but there is a normal daytime average ABPM (📖 Fig. 2.11).
- *White coat effect:* both clinic BP and ABPM are elevated, but clinic BP remains more elevated than the expected 10/5 or 12/7 mm Hg. This could be termed true hypertension with a white coat effect.

- *Masked hypertension:* normal office BP but high home or 24-h ABPMs (i.e. the reverse of white coat hypertension). It may be present in untreated people as a prelude to the onset of hypertension. No outcome evidence on the benefits of intervention for treating masked hypertension is currently available.

Indications for 24-h ABPM

- Borderline hypertension without evidence of TOD.
- Resistant hypertension.
- White coat hypertension (Fig. 2.11).
- Labile hypertension.
- Assessment of nocturnal dipping.
- Assessment of postural hypotension in symptomatic patients without overt postural changes.
- Autonomic failure.

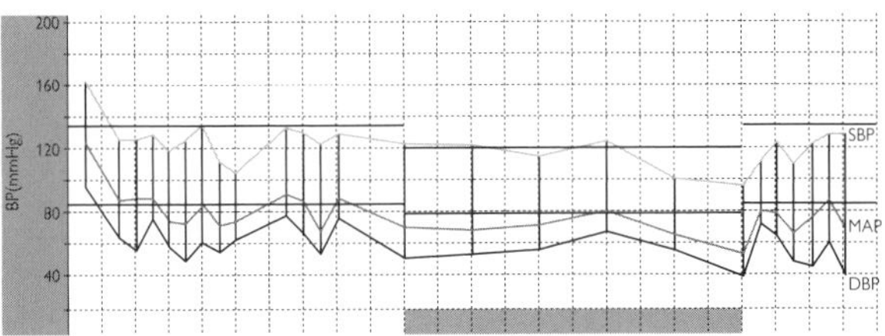

Fig. 2.11 A 24-h ABPM depicting the white coat effect. SBP, DBP, and mean arterial pressure (MAP) are labelled. Note the first reading is very high in the clinic but all the subsequent readings are entirely normal. There is also a normal diurnal variation in that the night-time readings dip as expected.

Reference

1. Automatic digital blood pressure devices for clinical use and also suitable for home/self assessment. Available at the BHS website: http://www.bhsoc.org/bp_monitors/automatic.stm

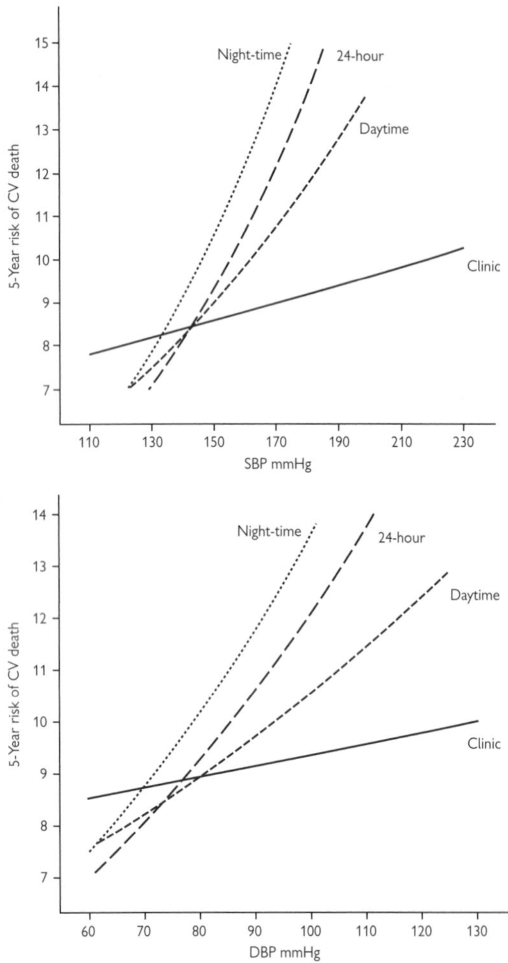

Fig. 2.12 Adjusted 5-year risk of cardiovascular death in the study cohort of 1,144 older patients for CBPM and ABPM. Using multiple Cox regression, the relative risk was calculated with adjustment for baseline characteristics including gender, age, presence of diabetes mellitus, history of cardiovascular events and smoking status. Five-year risks are expressed as number of deaths per 100 subjects. Reproduced from Burr ML *et al.* (2008). The value of ambulatory blood pressure in older adults: the Dublin outcome study. *Age and Ageing.* **37**:201–6, Oxford University Press.

Echocardiography

Echocardiography (echo) is a non-invasive, non-radioactive, ultrasound-based tool that helps visualize the dynamic function and anatomical structure of the heart.

Two-dimensional (2D) echo has a few advantages over other investigations in the setting of hypertension. Primarily, it is a more reliable and sensitive method of assessing LVH than a standard 12-lead ECG.[1] This is particularly important in the setting of a patient with borderline or resistant hypertension when the decision to treat or not treat depends on the presence or absence of LVH. Similarly, the effectiveness of therapy can be assessed in terms of regression of LVH post-therapy. LVH, as already mentioned, is an independent risk factor for CV mortality above and beyond BP *per se*. Echo can also distinguish LVH due to HOCM from that due to hypertension—this is an important diagnostic point.

Echo can also estimate left ventricular mass using a variety of methods including M-mode and 2D imaging, and newer methods including contrast echo, three-dimensional (3D) echo, and cardiac MRI may improve this in the future. Additionally, in some patients the presence of a coarctation may be diagnosed using echo.

Left ventricular systolic function can be assessed using ejection fraction on 2D echo or fractional shortening on M-mode echo. Diastolic function is assessed using a number of methods, and in particular with tissue Doppler imaging.

In cases of Type A aortic dissection, visualization of the aortic root may occasionally be difficult—transoesophageal echo may help determine the type of dissection more readily.

Reference

1. Kannel WB (1972). Role of blood pressure in the development of congestive heart failure: The Framingham Study. *NEJM* **287**:781–7.

Prognosis and risk stratification

Hypertension is a strong risk factor for CVD—this is a continuous and graded association (📖 Fig. 2.13). However, there are other risk factors which multiply the absolute risk of developing CVD. Note the difference between absolute risk and lifetime risk (📖 Box 2.7). There is no point in estimating risk in those who have already suffered an event.

Box 2.7 Definition of risk terminology

- *Absolute risk*: the excess risk due to exposure to a specific hazard.
- *Lifetime risk*: the risk of developing a disease during an individual's lifetime or dying of the disease.

These risk factors may be inherited or acquired and therefore may be modified or not depending on the risk factor itself (Box 2.8).

Box 2.8 Risk factors for CVD

Inherited risk factors

- Age.
- Sex.
- Racial origin.
- Family history.
- Type 1 diabetes mellitus.

Acquired/modifiable risk factors

- BP.
- LDL cholesterol.
- Arterial stiffness.
- Smoking.
- BMI.
- Pulse pressure.
- Exercise.
- LVH.
- Microalbuminuria.

To quantify risk, there are a number of multivariate risk formulas that require discrete information about the individual patient that can be input to work out an individual's risk of developing CVD. These are only to be used on untreated patients and are based on large populations (primarily Caucasian) which mean that they are not necessarily representative of other populations (Box 2.9).

The Joint British Societies (JBS) have issued recommendations on preventing CVD, including a CVD risk prediction chart, based on the Framingham database (📖 see Figs. 2.14 and 2.15).

Box 2.9 Risk calculators

- Framingham coronary prediction score sheets.
- Dundee risk disk.
- Sheffield tables.
- PROCAM risk.
- Joint British Societies (JBS) guidelines.

These charts have been primarily designed for 1° prevention and are an aid to making clinical decisions about when to intervene on lifestyle and whether to use antihypertensives, lipid-lowering medication, or aspirin. Patients with persistently elevated BP >160/100mmHg with TOD should have their BP treated, irrespective of calculated risk.

For patients from the Indian subcontinent, assume that the risk is 1.5 × higher than that predicted from the charts. Treatment is recommended if the 10-year CVD risk for the individual is ≥20%.

The charts are not for individuals who have:

- Overt evidence of CHD.
- Familial hypercholesterolaemia or other dyslipidaemias.
- Chronic renal dysfunction.
- Diabetes mellitus.
- Age <35 years.

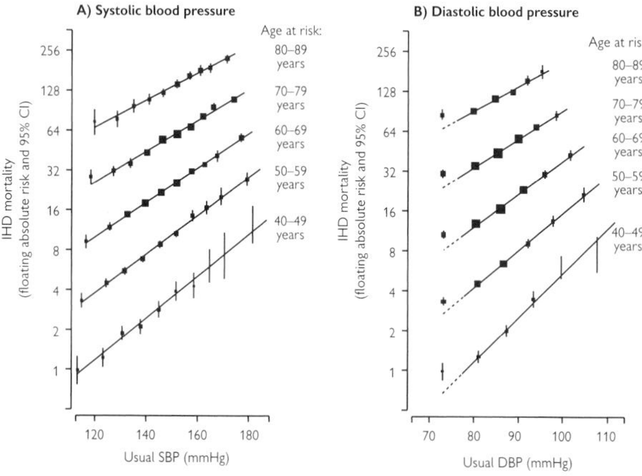

Fig. 2.13 The relationship between the risk of mortality from ischaemic heart disease and blood pressure in a meta-analysis of >1 million subjects. The data are similar for stroke. Redrawn from Lewington S, *et al.* (2002). Age-specific relevance of usual blood pressure to vascular mortality: a meta-analysis of individual data for one million adults in 61 prospective studies. *Lancet* **360**:1903–13 © 2002, with permission from Elsevier.

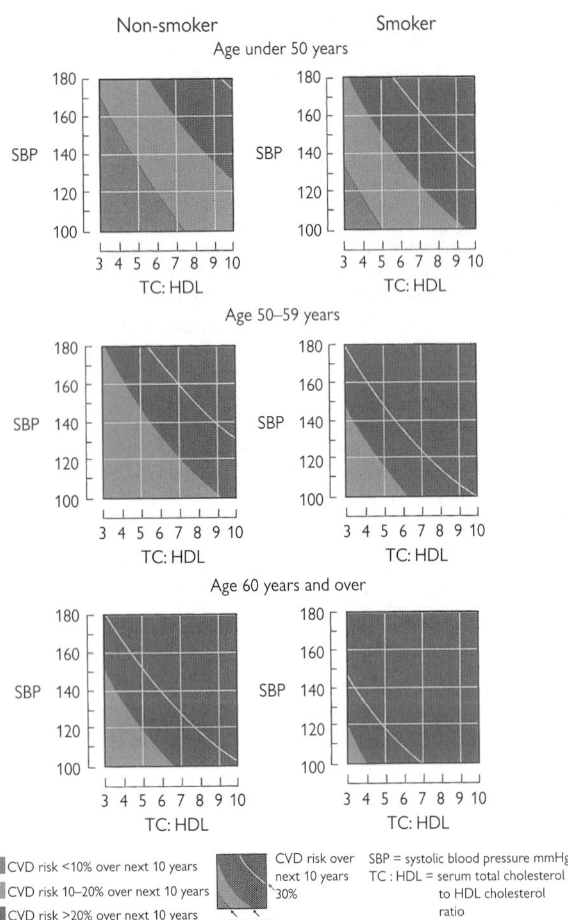

Fig. 2.14 JBS guidelines on CVD risk prediction for non-diabetic men. Reproduced with permission from the University of Manchester.

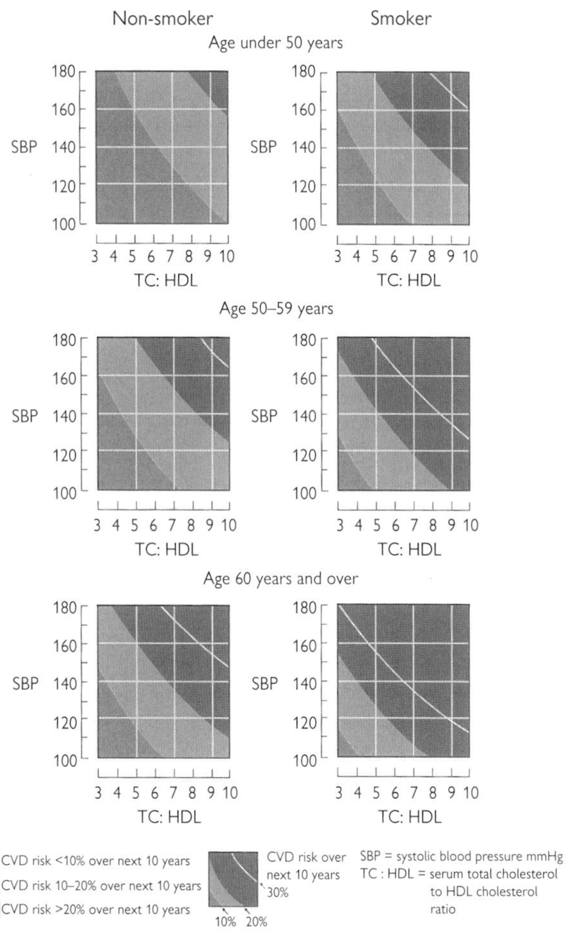

Fig. 2.15 JBS guidelines on CVD risk prediction for non-diabetic women. Reproduced with permission from the University of Manchester.

Non-pharmacological management: background

- Non-pharmacological management remains a mainstay in the management of all individuals—whether hypertensive or not, with or without end-organ damage.
- The positive benefit of these interventions has a role to play in preventing, ameliorating, and reducing the burden of CV risk factors across any risk groups.
- It engenders patients to take responsibility for their own health and should be recommended whether a patient is on or about to start pharmacological treatment, unless contraindicated by other concomitant conditions.
- Dietary alteration and exercise are the most obvious areas which may help reduce BP without drug therapy. The evidence for this stems from epidemiological data as discussed in 📖 Prevalence and incidence, p.50.
- Although the individual benefits of each intervention may appear modest at best, they may, in combination, be crucial—especially in the borderline hypertensive patient—to avoid pharmacological therapies. A summary of these effects are listed in 📖 Table 2.5.
- In addition, it is important to remember that some lifestyle interventions may not affect BP *per se* but have dramatic impact on CV risk, and are therefore crucial to the holistic management of the hypertensive patient. Examples include avoiding a high fat diet and smoking.
- In the Trials of Hypertension Prevention (TOHP I and II) study, the effect of lifestyle changes in people with high normal blood pressure was examined. Weight loss and sodium reduction significantly lowered BP but not stress/nutritional management. This translated in the longer term to a reduction in CV mortality and morbidity in those assigned to sodium reduction.[1]

Smoking

Whilst smoking causes a temporary rise in pressure, it has not been implicated in epidemiological studies with ↑ BP per se. In fact, there is an inverse relationship between smoking and ↑ BP. Nevertheless, smoking remains an important risk factor for the development of CVD and is therefore vital in the calculation of an individual's risk.

Smoking cessation is associated with a reduction in susceptibility to coronary events by nearly 50% and this can occur within a short time frame of 2 years. Risk of CV events is thought to normalize to a non-smoker's risk at 15 years post cessation.

Reference

1. Cook NR *et al.* (2007). Long term effects of dietary sodium reduction on cardiovascular disease outcomes: observational follow-up of the trials of hypertension prevention (TOHP). *BMJ* **334**(7599):885.

Table 2.5 Effects of lifestyle modification*

Intervention	Recommendation	Expected SBP reduction (range)
Weight reduction	Maintain ideal BMI (20–25kg/m^2)	5–10mmHg per 10kg weight loss
Diet	Consume diet rich in fruit, vegetables, and fibre, but low in fat	8–14mmHg
Reduced sodium intake	<100mmol/day (<6g of sodium chloride or <2.4g of sodium/day)	2–8mmHg
Physical activity	Regular aerobic physical activity, e.g. brisk walking for at least 30 min at least 5 days/week	4–9mmHg
Alcohol moderation	No more than 3 units/day in men; no more than 2 units/day in women	2–4mmHg

*Adapted from, US Department of Health and Human Services (2003) with permission. The JNC 7 Report. Source: The National Heart, Lung and Blood Institute (part of the National Institute of Health and the US Department of Health and Human Services)

Salt

Salt intake is closely linked to hypertension—the kidney is central to salt and water retention. Western populations currently consume at least 6–10 × more salt (~9–10g/day) than required, so it is not surprising that intervention to reduce this may have an effect. Most of this salt is from processed foods, cereals, meat, and milk (📖 Box 2.10).

The Dietary Approaches to Stop Hypertension (DASH) Trial was an intervention trial which showed a clear dose–response between the amount of Na^+ restriction and the level of BP achieved (📖 Fig. 2.16).[1] Meta-analysis of intervention trials indicate a reduction of 5/2.5mmHg in SBP and DBP with just a 50mmol reduction in Na^+ intake.[2]

A reduction in salt intake from 10g to 6g a day (current UK recommendations) theoretically could, via a reduction in BP, lead to a 16% reduction in stroke mortality and 12% reduction CHD mortality. This would theoretically prevent approximately 19,000 stroke and heart attack deaths in the UK each year and 2.6 million each year worldwide.[3] There are no interventional trials to prove this outcome.

Salt sensitivity also has a profound effect—most hypertensives are salt sensitive compared to their normotensive counterparts. There are also racial differences with more hypertensive people of African descent being salt sensitive than non-African hypertensives.

Box 2.10 Salt conversion

- 100mmol/day salt = 6g salt/day = ~2.3g Na^+/day = 100mmol/day Na^+.
- At steady state, urinary excretion of Na^+ = dietary intake, i.e. there is 100% bioavailability.

References

1. Sacks FM, *et al.* (2001). Effect on bloods pressure of reduced dietary sodium and the Dietary Approaches to Stop Hypertension (DASH) diet. *NEJM* **344**:3–10.
2. Law MR, *et al.* (1991). By how much does dietary salt reduction lower blood pressure? III – Analysis of data from trials of salt reduction. *BMJ* **302**:819–24.
3. Salt and blood pressure. Available at Consensus Action on Salt and Health (CASH) website: http://www.actiononsalt.org.uk/health/salt_and_health/blood_pressure.htm

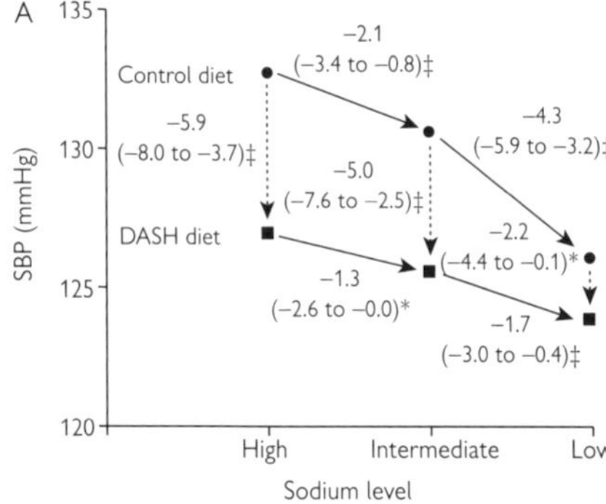

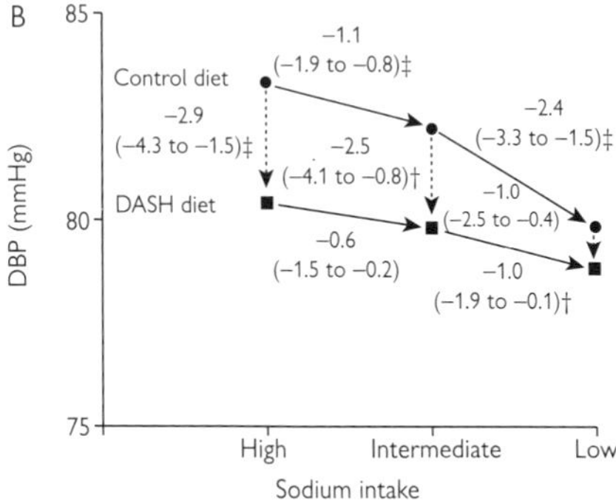

Fig. 2.16 Dose–response to reduced salt intake in the DASH study. Adapted with permission from Sacks FM, *et al.* (2001). Effect on bloods pressure of reduced dietary sodium and the Dietary Approaches to Stop Hypertension (DASH) diet. *NEJM* **344**:3–10, © 2001 Massachusetts Medical Society, all rights reserved.

Dietary intervention, weight loss, and exercise

Healthy diets

A diet low in saturated fats, high in fruits, vegetables, low-fat dairy products, fibre, and plant-derived grains and proteins is recommended, as is oily fish. Some of this is reflected in the recent UK Department of Health campaign for 5 portions of fruit a day ('5 A Day') to reduce the burden of CVD in the population.

There are no outcome data on how a healthy diet consisting of low fat, high fruit and vegetables reduces mortality or morbidity from CVD—however, vegetarians have lower BP than non-vegetarians in both population-based and clinical trials.

Fish-oil supplementation in large doses does lower BP by around 4/2mmHg. It has also been shown in meta-analyses that omega-3-polyunsaturated fatty acids and oily fish reduce CV mortality. (📖 See also Box 2.11.)

Weight loss and obesity

The likely beneficial effects of dietary interventions on BP may not be directly from the better diet but perhaps from the associated weight loss.

Obesity and hypertension co-exist within the metabolic syndrome—a combination of CV risk factors that include insulin resistance and dyslipidaemia. This is a phenomenon that is ↑ throughout the world—35% of the adult population in Europe is overweight whilst 18% are obese.

Every 10kg of excess weight is associated with a 3/2mmHg ↑ in BP suggesting a 12% ↑ in IHD and 24% ↑ in stroke. Weight loss is associated with a ↓ in BP—in a meta-analysis[1] of 24 randomized controlled trials (RCTs), a 5kg weight loss is associated with a 4/3mmHg ↓ in BP. Low calorie diets may ↓ SBP in some people by about 10mmHg.

Exercise

Regular aerobic exercise (30–60min, 3–5 ×/week) is recommended at all ages. The ↑ sedentary lifestyle of westernized populations (around 70% in the UK) means that the general CV fitness of the population is in decline. This predisposes to an ↑ burden of CVD especially in an ageing population subjected to unhealthy diets and rising levels of obesity.

A recent meta-analysis[2] of trials in both aerobic (72 trials) and resistance training (9 trials) revealed a fall in BP of 3/3mmHg mediated through a reduction in systemic vascular resistance and with positive effects on a variety of CV risk factors.

Box 2.11 Other dietary modifications

K^+ supplementation

There is some evidence to suggest K^+ supplementation may reduce BP by small amounts but there is no outcome data to support its widespread use.

Ca^{2+} supplementation

Apart from 1 review which showed a small benefit, there are no outcome data to suggest this has any effect on outcome.

Mg^{2+} supplementation

There are no data to support supplementation of Mg^{2+} in terms of BP or outcome, especially so in hypertensives.

References

1. Neter JE, *et al.* (2003). Influence of weight reduction on blood pressure: a meta-analysis of randomized controlled trials. *Hypertension* **42**:878–95.
2. Fagard RH and Cornelissen VA (2007). Effect of exercise on blood pressure control in hypertensive patients. *Eur J Cardiovasc Prev Rehabil* **14**:12–17.

Alcohol

There is a strong relationship between the pattern and quantity of alcohol intake and hypertension and CV mortality. Since World War I, it has been known that there is a graded relationship between alcohol intake and BP,[1] although other groups reported a J-shaped curve between overall mortality and alcohol—sometimes due to misclassification of occasional drinkers as non-drinkers. A 23-year follow-up study by Doll *et al.* (📖 see Fig. 2.17) has, however, proved it was J shaped—even after correcting for this difference—and for all-cause mortality as well as ischaemic heart disease.

In a study of >80,000 people in the USA, there was a linear relationship (in middle-aged white men drinking >2 daily drinks) of the number of drinks consumed per day and the level of BP.[2] Abstainers and light drinkers had lower levels of BP and drinkers who stopped drinking had a fall in BP. This correlation has been shown repeatedly in many other cross-sectional and epidemiological studies across wide populations and independent of other risk factors (📖 Fig. 2.18).

It is now thought that the 'French paradox' of reduced CHD despite moderate red wine intake may be due to the wine's effects on HDL cholesterol or antithrombotic effects.

Generally, non-drinkers should not be encouraged to start drinking, but drinkers should be advised to drink moderately whilst chronic alcoholics should be encouraged to abstain altogether.[3] A meta-analysis of 15 RCTs showed a modest reduction of 3/2mmHg in BP when alcohol reduction was reduced across a range of trials (📖 see Fig. 1.24).

References

1. Lian C (1915). L'alcoholisme, cause d'hypertension arterielle. *Bulletin de l'Academie de Medicine* **74**:525–8.
2. Klatsky AL, *et al.* (1977). Alcohol consumption and blood pressure. Kaiser-Permanente Multiphasic Health Examination data. *NEJM* **296**:1194–2000.
3. Klatsky AL (2007). Alcohol, cardiovascular diseases and diabetes mellitus. *Pharmacol Res* **55**:237–47.

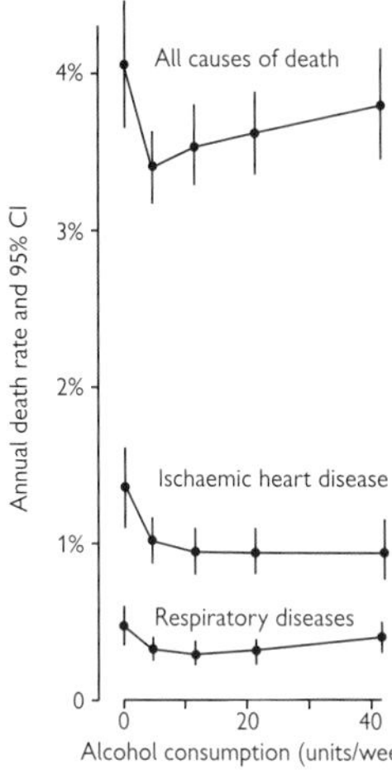

Fig. 2.17 The association between all-cause mortality and alcohol consumption is a J-shaped curve. Reproduced from Doll R, *et al.* (2005). Mortality in relation to alcohol consumption: a prospective study among male British doctors. *Int J Epidemiol* **34**:199–204, with permission from Oxford University Press.

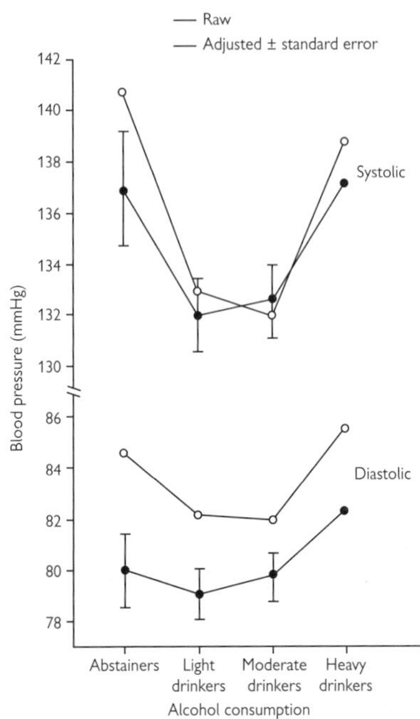

Fig. 2.18 Mean systolic and diastolic blood pressure (raw and adjusted for potential confounders) by alcohol consumption in men aged 35–64 years in Auckland, New Zealand, 1982. Reproduced from Jackson R, *et al.* (1985). Alcohol consumption and blood pressure. *American Journal of Epidemiology* **122**:1037–44, Oxford University Press.

Other methods

Acupuncture

Acupuncture, an ancient Chinese technique, was recently subjected to a single, blinded RCT in treated and untreated mild to moderate hypertensives.[1] Patients underwent a 6-week treatment course and were followed up at 6 months. This showed that there was a 5/3mmHg difference in ambulatory pressures initially, which then rose to pre-treatment levels at 6 months.

Another randomized trial (SHARP[2]) showed no difference in BP reduction between the acupuncture and sham groups. The obvious design problems are lack of an effective control and effective blinding of both the patient and administering therapist.

Breathing modulation devices

The US Food and Drug administration has approved a device which allows patients to modulate their breathing to music. The approval is for stress reduction and as an adjunct to hypertension management. This is based on preliminary evidence that the device may ameliorate BP. A series of studies have shown the potential for this device to reduce BP by retraining patients to breathe in relation to the music they hear. The mechanism is thought to be via a reduction in sympathetic activity utilizing slowed breathing.[3]

References

1. Flachskampf FA, *et al.* (2007). Randomized trial of acupuncture to lower blood pressure. *Hypertension* **115**:3121–9.
2. Macklin EA, *et al.* (2006). Stop Hypertension with acupuncture research (SHARP). *Hypertension* **48**:838–45.
3. Resperate http://www.resperate.com/us/discover/clinicalproof.aspx#peer_reviewed_articles

Pharmacological management: background

Drug therapy is indicated when the benefit of therapy outweighs risks. Careful estimation of this risk should be undertaken as already described, especially when encountering a borderline patient.

Drug therapy does not obviate the need for non-pharmacological methods (📖 see Non-pharmacological management, pp.88–96). Additionally, therapy should include anything to reduce all risk factors, not just BP *per se*.

The drug classes to treat ↑ BP are discussed in 📖 Chapter 7. One major issue, which has been resolved to some extent, is whether different drugs are more effective than others in reducing CV mortality.

Drug choice

The ALLHAT[1] trial demonstrated little difference between the diuretic, calcium-channel antagonist (CCA), and ACEI regimens on outcome, thereby answering this question. The α-blocker arm was, however, discontinued early due to the presence of ankle oedema which was thought to represent worsening heart failure.

The ASCOT[2] trial, however, suggests that newer drug regimens (ACEI and CCA) fare better than older drug regimens (β-blocker and diuretic) in all-cause mortality, stroke (by 25%), and coronary events (by 15%). However, the 1° endpoint of non-fatal MI was not statistically significant between the groups. ASCOT also clearly demonstrated the need for multiple risk factor management to reduce CV risk effectively.

What remains unclear is the role of β-blockers in the management of hypertension—it is certainly not a first-line recommended drug class for hypertension except in young people or in pregnancy.

References

1. ALLHAT Officers and Coordinators (2002). Major outcomes in high-risk patients randomized to angiotensin-converting enzyme inhibitor or calcium channel blocker vs. diuretic: the Antihypertensive and Lipid Lowering Treatment to prevent Heart Attack Trial (ALLHAT). *JAMA* **288**:2981–97.
2. Dahlöf B, *et al.* (2005). Prevention of cardiovascular events with an antihypertensive regimen of amlodipine adding perindopril as required versus atenolol adding bendroflumethiazide as required, in the Anglo-Scandinavian Cardiac Outcomes Trial-Blood Pressure Lowering Arm (ASCOT-BPLA): a multicentre randomised controlled trial. *Lancet* **366**:895–906.

Compliance

Compliance refers to the patient's adherence to their prescribed drug regimen. It represents a major problem in medicine and in hypertension in particular, primarily because hypertension is generally asymptomatic and drug therapy inevitably causes side effects.

There are many factors which worsen and improve compliance; these are listed in 📖 Box 2.12.

Box 2.12 Factors affecting compliance

Factors causing non-compliance

- Asymptomatic disease.
- Cost of drug therapy.
- Patient's perception surrounding risks of drug therapy.
- Patient's perception regarding drug effectiveness.
- Drug side effect profile.
- Forgetfulness.
- Poor labelling.
- Poor packaging.
- Polypharmacy.
- Social factors.

Factors to improve compliance

- Clear explanation of risk/benefit arguments.
- Patient empowerment in decision-making process.
- Informed choices through education.
- Individualization of therapy.
- Concordance (patient and doctor agree on regimen).
- Simplify drug regimen.
- Regular contact and continuing supervision.
- Home monitoring.

Monitoring compliance

It is possible to monitor compliance through a variety of manoeuvres including:

- Patient request for repeat prescriptions at appropriate intervals.
- Drug accountability.
- Directly observed drug therapy.
- Monitoring drug levels (for certain drugs only).

Stepped care versus combination therapy

Stepped care refers to the current practice within national guidelines which advocate using the lowest possible dose of an initial drug and then titrating this compound up the dose–response curve (as tolerated by the patient) to the maximum dose before then commencing a second-line therapy. Its aim is to reduce polypharmacy and improve compliance.

However, improving the efficacy of the drug by ↑ the dose is in many ways counterintuitive as it moves in a direction which is more likely to cause more side effects, and therefore worsen the side-effect profile of the drug, thereby reducing patient satisfaction and ↑ the risk of non-compliance.

Combination therapy refers to using low doses of 2 agents, either in a single pill or in quick succession as add-on therapy. This usually results in a greater clinical efficacy with reduced side effects compared to uptitration. This, may in part, be due to synergism, or may be due to the offsetting of 1 side effect by the action of the complementary drug. Combination therapy therefore offers the clinician the opportunity to maximize clinical efficacy and minimize adverse events to the benefit of the patient.

This concept has allowed for safer fixed-dose combination therapies to be developed. This not only enhances clinical efficacy but simplifies the drug regimen for the patient, and similarly the practical aspects of prescribing for the clinician. In an era where it is clear that the lower the BP, the lower the incident risk, it is probably time that most guidelines move towards a combination therapy system.

Targets and evidence basis

The treatment thresholds to start antihypertensive therapy are different to the treatment targets.

The BHS recommend initiation[1] of antihypertensive therapy in:

- Those with BP ≥160/100mmHg persistently on ≥2 occasions.
- In diabetics, renal impairment, established CVD, TOD, or those with a CVD risk ≥20% *and* SBP 140–159mmHg and/or DBP 90–99mmHg.

The recommended treatment goals or targets are:

- SBP <140mmHg, DBP <85mmHg in non-diabetic hypertensives but the minimum acceptable level of control is <150/90mmHg (Audit Standard).
- SBP <130mm Hg, DBP <80mmHg in diabetic hypertensives, Audit Standard is <140/80mmHg.
- Main benefit comes from BP achieved, not the drug used.
- Low-dose aspirin and statin therapy should be used to reduce CVD risk—statins for all hypertensives with CVD, CVD risk ≥ 20% irrespective of baseline cholesterol.
- Good glycaemic control in diabetics with HbA1c <7%.

Note that the JBS guidelines for target BP are based primarily on the HOT study.[2] Efforts are currently underway in the USA to study whether the benefits of lowering the threshold for target SBP to <120mmHg in all non-diabetic patients may also be beneficial (Systolic Blood Pressure Intervention Trial—SPRINT).

Diabetics are considered coronary equivalents since their risks of coronary disease are ↑ by virtue of their diabetes alone. Intensive lowering of BP in diabetics, where possible, retards progression to microvascular as well as macrovascular complications (📖 see Diabetes, pp.196–199)

References

1. Williams B, *et al.* (2004) Guidelines for the management of hypertension: report of the fourth working party of the British Hypertension Society, 2004-BHS IV. *J Hum Hypertens* **18**:139–85.
2. Hansson L, *et al.* for the HOT Study Group (1998). Effects of intensive blood pressure lowering and low dose aspirin in patients with hypertension: principal results of the Hypertension Optimal Treatment (HOT) randomized trial. *Lancet* **351**:1755–62.

Treatment algorithms

Treatment guidelines are a relatively new method of implementing evidence base into day-to-day practice. The beneficial effect of BP reduction, albeit well known, remains suboptimal throughout the world.

Guidelines are available at international, national, and local levels. Whilst they do not all conform to a similar pattern, nor provide the same information, they should be evidence-based and adapt to the ever changing information available. Many guidelines are based on socio-economic factors that predicate certain treatments over others, whilst others depend on the nature of the health system in that country.

The algorithm for essential hypertension reproduced here (📖 Fig. 2.19) is from our local clinic guidelines which are based on the 'ACD' rule developed in Cambridge, UK (📖 Fig. 2.20). This was formally adopted by the BHS and the National Institute of Health and Clinical Excellence (NICE) in the UK and forms the basis of the current Joint BHS–NICE guidelines (📖 Fig. 2.21). The same applies to the algorithm for resistant hypertension (📖 Fig. 2.22) in the next section 📖 Resistant hypertension, p.106.

The most important criterion is BP reduction, irrespective of the type of drug used. However, β-blockers should be avoided in the elderly, especially those with ISH. They may be used in the younger patient although we would avoid the older non-selective agent such as atenolol. These agents also ↑ the risk of developing diabetes when used in conjunction with thiazide diuretics, especially in high-risk groups.

Tolerability, availability, and cost form the cornerstone of therapy and we would recommend the ACD guidelines, especially if there is no specific indication for a particular class of agent in a particular patient.

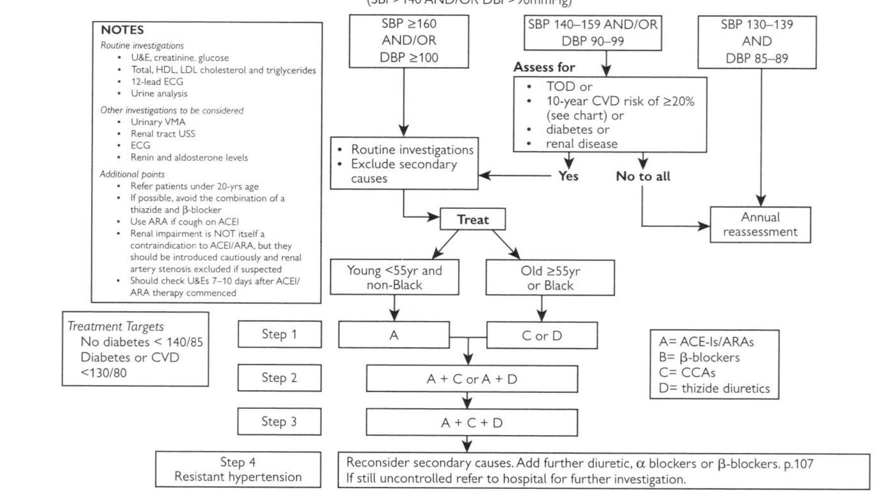
Treatment guideline for essential hypertension
(SBP>140 AND/OR DBP>90mmHg)
NOTES
Routine investigations
• U&E, creatinine, glucose
• Total, HDL, LDL cholesterol and triglycerides
• 12-lead ECG
• Urine analysis
Other investigations to be considered
• Urinary VMA
• Renal tract USS
• ECG
• Renin and aldosterone levels
Additional points
• Refer patients under 20-yrs age
• If possible, avoid the combination of a thiazide and β-blocker
• Use ARA if cough on ACEI
• Renal impairment is NOT itself a contraindication to ACEI/ARA, but they should be introduced cautiously and renal artery stenosis excluded if suspected
• Should check U&Es 7–10 days after ACEI/ARA therapy commenced
SBP ≥160 AND/OR DBP ≥100
SBP 140–159 AND/OR DBP 90–99
SBP 130–139 AND DBP 85–89
Assess for
• TOD or
• 10-year CVD risk of ≥20% (see chart) or
• diabetes or
• renal disease
• Routine investigations
• Exclude secondary causes
Yes
No to all
Annual reassessment
Treat
Young <55yr and non-Black
Old ≥55yr or Black
Treatment Targets
No diabetes < 140/85
Diabetes or CVD <130/80
Step 1
A
C or D
Step 2
A + C or A + D
Step 3
A + C + D
A= ACE-Is/ARAs
B= β-blockers
C= CCAs
D= thizide diuretics
Step 4
Resistant hypertension
Reconsider secondary causes. Add further diuretic, α blockers or β-blockers. p.107
If still uncontrolled refer to hospital for further investigation.

Fig. 2.19 Algorithm for management of essential hypertension.

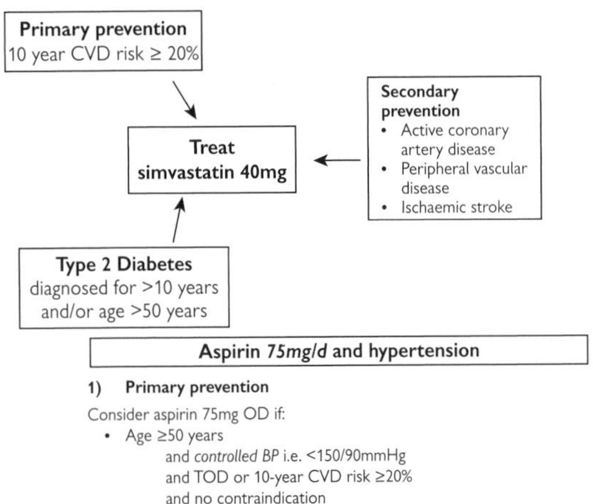

Aspirin *75mg/d* and hypertension

1) **Primary prevention**

Consider aspirin 75mg OD if:

- Age ≥50 years
  and *controlled BP* i.e. <150/90mmHg
  and TOD or 10-year CVD risk ≥20%
  and no contraindication

2) **Secondary prevention**

Such patients should already be on aspirin, unless there is a specific contraindication.

Fig. 2.20 Cambridge guidelines for 2° prevention.

Choosing drugs for patients newly diagnosed with hypertension

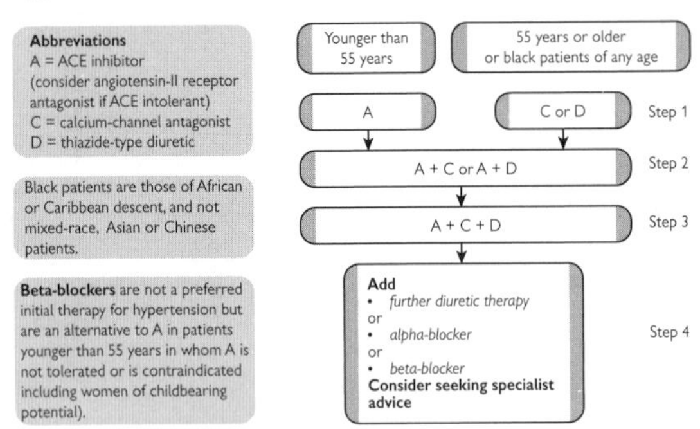

Fig. 2.21 Joint NICE–BHS guidelines on hypertension management.

Resistant hypertension

- Resistant hypertension is defined as a BP >140/90mmHg despite ≥ 3 antihypertensives.
- There are a variety of reasons that may underlie this and these are summarized in Box 2.13.
- There is little evidence to guide the physician in this area. More studies are required—the BHS will be launching a series of studies to examine this in greater detail shortly, under its Pathway Project.
- In the interim, we suggest following the algorithm as described in 📖 Fig. 2.22.
- All patients with resistant hypertension, should, after exclusion of artificial causes, be considered for investigation of 2° causes; in particular, hyperaldosteronism or renovascular disease, by a specialist.
- The role of ↑ diuretics, particularly aldosterone antagonists, in a cohort of these resistant patients, as effective antihypertensives, was recently reported in the ASCOT study.[1]

Box 2.13 Causes of resistant hypertension

Artificial
- Poor technique—cuff sizes.
- Lack of compliance.
- Non-concordance.
- Inadequate therapy.
- Age-related arterial stiffness—pseudohypertension.

True resistance
- Concomitant medication.
- White coat effect.
- Concomitant risk factors—obesity, alcohol excess, sleep apnoea, stress.
- Physiology—volume overload, baroreflex failure.
- 2° causes.
- Hereditary causes.

Reference

1. Chapman N, *et al.* (2007). Effect of spironolactone on blood pressure in subjects with resistant hypertension. *Hypertension* **49**:839–45.

Treatment algorithm for resistant hypertension (renin-based protocol)
(SBP>140 **AND/OR** DBP>85mmHg on 3 drugs)

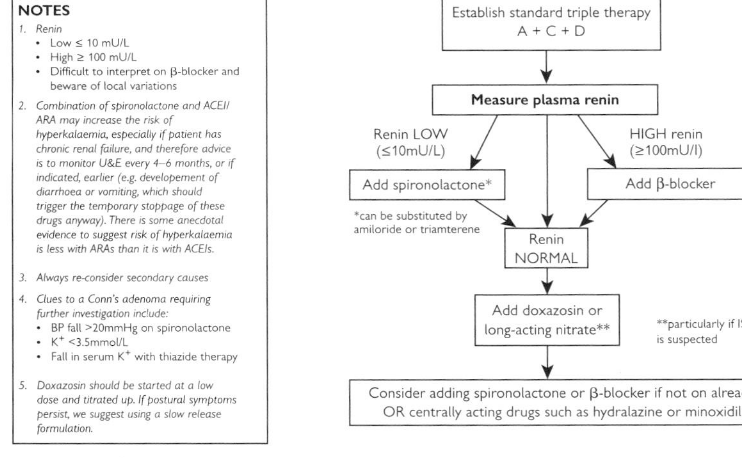
Establish standard triple therapy
A + C + D
Measure plasma renin
Renin LOW
(≤10mU/L)
HIGH renin
(≥100mU/l)
Add spironolactone*
Add β-blocker
*can be substituted by amiloride or triamterene
Renin NORMAL
Add doxazosin or long-acting nitrate**
**particularly if ISH is suspected
Consider adding spironolactone or β-blocker if not on already OR centrally acting drugs such as hydralazine or minoxidil
NOTES
1. Renin
• Low ≤ 10 mU/L
• High ≥ 100 mU/L
• Difficult to interpret on β-blocker and beware of local variations
2. Combination of spironolactone and ACEI/ARA may increase the risk of hyperkalaemia, especially if patient has chronic renal failure, and therefore advice is to monitor U&E every 4–6 months, or if indicated, earlier (e.g. developement of diarrhoea or vomiting, which should trigger the temporary stoppage of these drugs anyway). There is some anecdotal evidence to suggest risk of hyperkalaemia is less with ARAs than it is with ACEIs.
3. Always re-consider secondary causes
4. Clues to a Conn's adenoma requiring further investigation include:
• BP fall >20mmHg on spironolactone
• K+ <3.5mmol/L
• Fall in serum K+ with thiazide therapy
5. Doxazosin should be started at a low dose and titrated up. If postural symptoms persist, we suggest using a slow release formulation.

Fig. 2.22 Algorithm for management of resistant hypertension.

Hypertensive emergencies

The terminology here is crucial—there is a lot of confusion between the terms 'malignant hypertension', 'accelerated hypertension', 'hypertensive urgencies', and 'emergencies'.

It is perhaps best to use the terms 'accelerated phase hypertension' and 'hypertensive emergencies' only. The other terminology only adds to confusion about what requires immediate, urgent, or a more laissez faire approach to therapy (as in chronic hypertension). Both accelerated phase hypertension and hypertensive emergencies usually present with symptoms, unlike chronic hypertension.

Definitions

Accelerated phase hypertension is an abrupt rise in BP (sometimes with DBP ≥120mmHg), associated with retinal haemorrhages (± papilloedema) and occasionally proteinuria—which, if left untreated, can lead to a CV event (stroke, MI), renal failure, or blindness. This requires treatment to reduce BP over days to weeks using oral antihypertensive therapies, i.e. they need urgent but not immediate treatment. They should be followed-up closely. It commonly occurs in males, people of black descent, or in pre-existing hypertensives.

Hypertensive emergencies refer to a life-threatening situation wherein a severe, uncontrolled BP is associated with acute impairment of an organ system, e.g. aortic dissection, cardiac failure, hypertensive encephalopathy (or seizures), an acute stroke, eclampsia, phaeochromocytoma crisis, microangiopathic haemolytic anaemia, and so on. This requires BP to be brought down over minutes to hours in a controlled manner, usually using intravenous (IV) antihypertensives in an Intensive Care or Coronary Care Unit.

Hypertensive emergencies may present with or without changes associated with accelerated phase hypertension (i.e. there may or may not be papilloedema/retinal haemorrhages). The same is true vice versa. Patients with an elevated BP level without either should be defined as having 'severe uncontrolled hypertension'.

Pathophysiology of accelerated phase and hypertensive emergencies

This is not well understood—a rise in systemic vascular resistance due to loss of normal autoregulation results in progressive endothelial dysfunction leading to fibrinoid necrosis and intimal proliferation. Alternatively, there may be up-regulation of the renin–angiotensin system causing ↑ BP, a pressure natriuresis, and further release of vasoconstrictors which perpetuate a cycle of ↑ BP.

The aetiology is similar to that of hypertension in general—either essential or 2° to the known causes of hypertension—but it is perhaps worthwhile excluding a phaeochromocytoma, at least with urine screening tests in all these patients.

Epidemiology

It is thought to be prevalent in ~1% of hypertensives, although more effective and prompt therapy as soon as hypertension is diagnosed means that this is now falling rapidly in modern societies. It has an incidence of 2 per 100,000 cases per annum with a M:F ratio of 2:1.

Management of hypertensive emergencies

The management of a true hypertensive emergency should be on a high dependency unit, e.g. Intensive Care or Coronary Care. The aims are to safely and effectively reduce BP in a timely manner whilst observing for any change to the patient on a regular basis. Generally, short-acting, titratable antihypertensives are used intravenously to achieve this in a controlled manner.

Precipitous drops in BP can be catastrophic and should therefore be avoided. Careful monitoring and regular medical reviews are paramount to ensure proper management.

Aortic dissection

Type A dissection (which extends to the aortic root) usually requires medical *and* surgical management to repair the aortic root. Type B dissection requires medical management only, although endovascular repair and vascular surgery is sometimes indicated to protect vital organs, e.g. kidneys, limbs, etc.

The aim is to reduce SBP to 110mmHg and to reduce heart rate. Agents such as IV labetalol are recommended.

Labetalol is an α_1 and non-selective β antagonist with a $t_{1/2}$ of 5.5h. It has an onset of action within 2–5min. It may reduce heart rate but maintains cardiac output. Usual doses are a bolus dose (up to 50mg) over at least 1min or infusion at 2mg/min to a total dose of 200mg.

Hypertensive heart failure

This should be treated as left ventricular failure with IV nitrates and loop diuretics. IV sodium nitroprusside may also be used (📖 see Sodium nitroprusside, p.235). The dose is 10–15mcg/min, ↑ every 5–10min (usual range 10–200mcg/min) for a maximum of 3 days.

Hypertensive encephalopathy

This is rare but can present with neurological symptoms, seizures or coma (📖 see Colour plates 7 and 8). Diagnosis may be confirmed on MRI or CT. Management is with IV sodium nitroprusside, GTN, or labetalol. Seizures should be controlled with IV agents as per usual.

For sodium nitroprusside, the usual dose is 0.5–1.5mcg/kg/min, ↑ slowly to 0.5–8mcg/kg/min (lower if on other antihypertensives). It should be stopped if there is an unsatisfactory response to maximum dose at 10min. The aim is to reduce MAP by about 20% or to a DBP of ~100mmHg (whichever is greater) over 1h. Beware the patient with a cerebral ischaemic event—it is usual for a transient rise in BP—where the penumbra is hypoperfused during the infarct, and may be more so if IV anti-hypertensive therapy is used to lower pressure further (📖 Fig. 2.23).

Severe pre-eclampsia or eclampsia

This should be managed on a maternity ward; the main intervention is to delivery the fetus. The medical management includes intraveouns magnesium sulphate and control of BP using hydralazine or labetalol (📖 see Pregnancy: pre-eclampsia p.190).

Phaeochromocytoma crisis

This is one hypertensive emergency where β-blockade is contraindicated as it could worsen the hypertension via unopposed α-mediated vasoconstriction. Phentolamine IV, a rapid acting α-adrenergic antagonist, is the drug of choice.

Management of accelerated hypertension

- This should be directed at reducing BP over days to weeks. Oral agents are generally preferred. β-blockers or long-acting CCAs should be used as 1st-line agents.
- Short-acting CCAs (e.g. buccal nifedipine) should *not* be used as they may cause precipitous drops in BP, resulting in a CV event (e.g. stroke).
- ACEIs and ARAs may also cause precipitous drops in BP in the accelerated phase patient whose hypertension is being driven by renin. This may be evidenced by hypokalaemia on admission or other clues as mentioned in 📖 Examination, p.62.

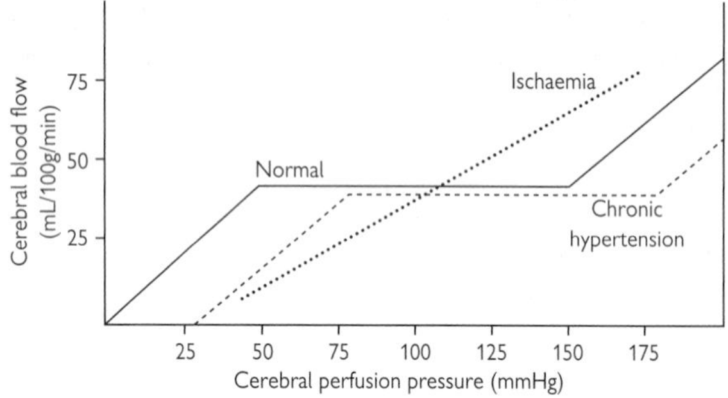

Fig. 2.23 Cerebral perfusion pressure is altered in chronic hypertension and cerebral ischaemia, so sudden drops in BP may worsen ischaemia in cerebral infarction.

Chapter 3

Specific investigations for secondary hypertension

Introduction

As discussed in Chapter 2, there may be clues from the history and examination or basic investigations which suggest a 2° cause of hypertension. In such cases, it will be necessary to then screen using non-invasive followed by invasive investigations to confirm these causes biochemically, and finally to confirm this with imaging.

The indications for these tests may vary from centre to centre. It is important to understand the details regarding how these tests are performed in the local laboratory as this may influence the sensitivity and specificity for diagnosis. A broad idea of this is provided in this chapter although these may not approximate the true sensitivity and specificity for your local laboratory.

Urine catecholamines and metanephrines

Catecholamines are metabolized to metanephrine and VMA which are then excreted in the urine (Fig. 3.1).

3 × 24-h urine collections for urinary VMA or catecholamines have been the standard screening test for phaeochromocytoma for many years. However, urinary metanephrines and normetanephrines (NMNs) may give better results. A recent retrospective analysis in Glasgow confirmed this in a series of 159 tests done (with 25 cases subsequently confirmed).[1] The results are shown in Box 3.1 (also see Phaeochromocytoma, p.152).

Box 3.1 Sensitivity and specificity of screening tests for phaeochromocytoma

	Sensitivity (%)	*Specificity (%)*
Urinary free metadrenalines	100	94
Urinary catecholamines	84	99
Urinary VMA	72	96
Plasma catecholamines	76	88

In general, these tests do not give an idea of the size or location of the phaeochromocytoma. They are useful screening tools and reasonably cheap, so may be used as a test in all new patients and those with resistant hypertension as a matter of routine. The pitfalls in diagnosis include an incomplete (i.e. <24-h) collection and false positives due to concomitant medications (Box 3.2).

Box 3.2 Drugs which cause false positive urine tests for phaeochromocytoma

- Acetaminophen.
- Alcohol.
- Aminophylline, theophylline.
- Amphetamines.
- Appetite suppressants.
- Caffeine.
- Clonidine.
- Diuretics.
- Epinephrine.
- Insulin.
- Lithium.
- Nicotine.
- Salicylates.
- Steroids.
- Tricyclics.
- Vasodilators.

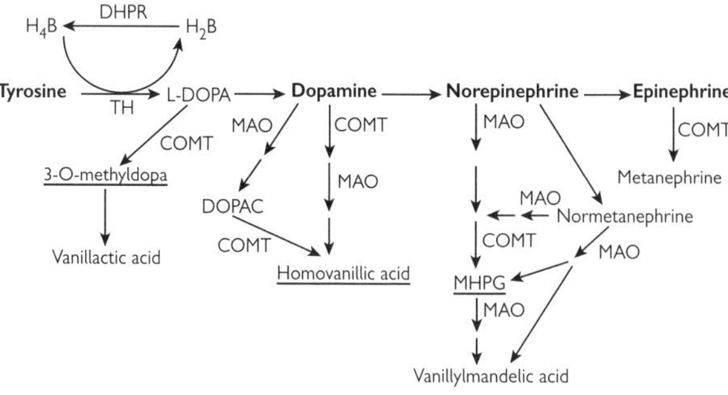

Fig. 3.1 Catecholamine metabolism.

Reference

1. Boyle JG, *et al.* (2007). Comparison of diagnostic accuracy of urinary free metanephrines, vanillyl mandelic acid, and catecholamines and plasma catecholamines for diagnosis of pheochromocytoma. *J Clin Endocrinol Metab* **92**:4602–8.

Plasma catecholamines and metanephrines

Plasma noradrenaline and adrenaline (i.e. catecholamines) may be measured in cases where there is a suspicion of a phaeochromocytoma. This may be in conjunction with urinary metanephrines and NMNs or VMAs, or in cases where the diagnosis is strongly suspected but the urine tests are negative. However, although rare, it is unlikely that an intermittently secreting phaeochromocytoma will be diagnostic on plasma catecholamines unless these are obtained during an episode.

This is usually done by the high performance liquid chromatography electrochemical (HPLC-EC) technique (📖 Fig. 3.2). This well established assay relies on the extraction of catecholamines from plasma and then separation on the basis of their retention patterns within a column in a C18 column. A non-naturally occurring catecholamine (dihydroxybenzylamine, DHBA) is used as an internal standard to correct for any losses during the extraction.

Additionally, plasma metanephrines and NMNs have been shown to be even better predictors, especially in patients with intermittently secreting tumours (presumably due to continued metabolization of catecholamines). This has been reported to provide a sensitivity of 97% and specificity of between 92–96%.[1,2] Reference intervals in the local laboratory should ensure the primacy of sensitivity over specificity.

Improvements in the analytical technology (liquid chromatography with tandem mass spectrophotometry, radioimunnoassay, ELISA, etc.) are already having a major impact on the diagnostic rates obtainable. The clinician should also consider the possibility false negatives in patients with either very small tumours or those which do not produce catecholamines (e.g. dopamine)—where measurement of other markers such as plasma dopamine or methoxytyramine may be important.[2]

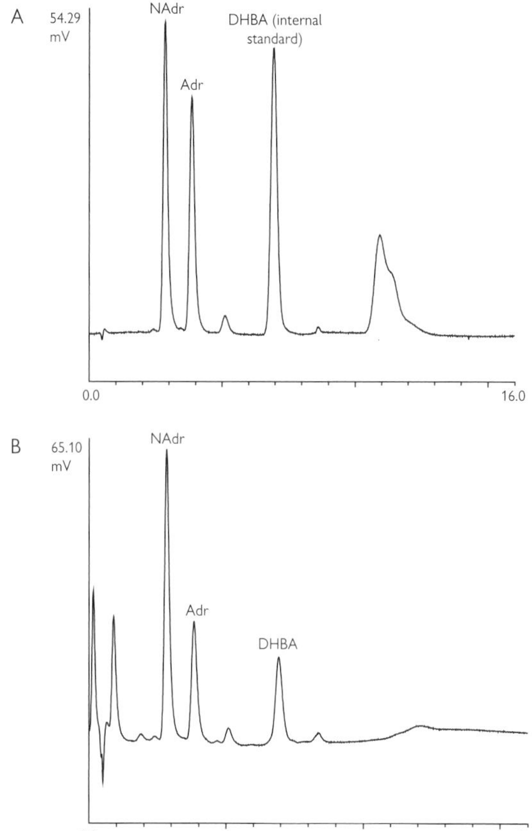

Fig. 3.2 HPLC assays for catecholamines. A comparison is made to the internal standard, normal (A), and a patient with adrenal phaeochromocytoma secreting noradrenaline (B).

References

1. Eisenhofer G, *et al.* (1999). Plasma metanephrine and normetanephrine for detecting phaeochromocytoma in Von Hippel Lindau disease and multiple endocrine neoplasia type 2. *NEJM* **340**:1872–9.
2. Eisenhofer G, *et al.* (2008). Current progress and future challenges in the biochemical diagnosis and treatment of pheochromocytomas and paragangliomas. *Hormone Metab Res* **40**:329–37.

Dynamic testing

These are tests which are performed to unmask or rule out the presence of a true phaeochromocytoma or paraganglionoma.

Provocation tests are performed when there are normal baseline results in someone who is thought to have a high clinical suspicion for a phaeochromocytoma. Suppression tests may be performed to establish that borderline baseline results are truly due to a true phaeochromocytoma or paraganglionoma (📖 see Box 3.3).

The provocation tests have gone out of fashion—mainly because:
- They may provoke a hypertensive crisis requiring phentolamine therapy.
- Poor sensitivity.
- More modern methods of measuring activity are available, e.g. urinary and plasma metanephrines which are far more sensitive.

Box 3.3 Provocation and suppression tests for suspected phaeochromocytomas and paraganglionomas

Provocation tests
- Histamine test.
- Tyramine test.
- Glucagon test.

Suppression tests
- Clonidine test.
- Pentolinium test.

Clonidine suppression test

Suppression tests tend to be used in those patients with borderline biochemistry for catecholamines but where the clinical suspicion is high (plasma noradrenaline/norepinephrine (NE) 500–2000ng/L (2.9–11.8nmol/L) or if plasma NE + E is 1000–2000ng/L (5.9–11.8nmol/L). They should not be used in patients with severe coronary or cerebrovascular disease or in those with hypotension.

Clonidine is an old antihypertensive agent which works as a direct agonist at the presynaptic α2-adrenergic receptor in the brain, thereby reducing cardiac output and systemic resistance and BP. It also inhibits noradrenaline release: this forms the basis of its use as a suppression test[1] (like pentolinium) for diagnosing phaeochromocytomas. The procedure is described in Box 3.4.

Box 3.4 Procedure

- Patient lays supine (having emptied bladder), IV cannula inserted and flushed.
- Rest for 30min.
- Measure BP and pulse.
- A blood sample is obtained for plasma NE (or NMN) from the cannula and recorded as the baseline sample. Store each sample on ice until centrifugation.
- Administer clonidine 0.3mg PO (note time).
- Patient remains supine, resting quietly. Further samples for plasma NE (or NMN) are then taken at 60, 120, and 180min.

A 50% reduction is quoted to be the expected suppression of NE from baseline in patients without a phaeochromocytoma. A positive response[2] is defined as 1 of either:

- Plasma NE >500ng/L (2.9nmol/L).
- Plasma NE >500ng/L and Δ plasma NE <50% (specificity 98%, sensitivity 67%).
- Plasma NMN >112ng/L and Δ plasma NMN <40% (specificity 100%, sensitivity 96%).

There is also usually no haemodynamic change in phaeochromocytoma patients but a ↓ in BP is seen in patients with essential hypertension or anxious patients.

There is a higher false-positive rate in patients on tricyclic antidepressants which should be omitted (depending on their $t_{1/2}$) and those with borderline NE values. The advantage is that it can be given orally. Clonidine suppresses normal levels of NE (at baseline) but not epinephrine; it is also long acting therefore the patient may remain hypotensive for hours (hence best to omit ß-blockers, diuretics and other antihypertensives, antidepressants) and may require overnight admission.

References

1. Bravo EL, *et al.* (1981). Clonidine suppression test: a useful aid in the diagnosis of phaeochromocytoma. *NEJM* **305**:623–6.
2. Eisenhofer G, *et al.* (2003). Biochemical diagnosis of pheochromocytoma: how to distinguish true from false-positive test results. *J Clin Endocrinol Metab* **88**:2656–66.

Pentolinium suppression test

This is usually performed to confirm the diagnosis of a phaeochromocytoma. Catecholamines (NE or Epinephrine) are released from adrenergic nerve endings by preganglionic cholinergic nerves. Pentolinium is a ganglion blocking agent which binds to the acetylcholine receptor, thereby preventing catecholamine release—hence its potential use as a suppression test.[1] Therefore failure to suppress NE or Epinephrine adequately after injection with pentolinium suggests autonomous secretion by a tumour, i.e. a phaeochromocytoma. The procedure is described in Box 3.5.

Box 3.5 Procedure

- Patient lays supine (having emptied bladder), IV cannula inserted and flushed.
- Rest for 30min before the next sample (for plasma NE or Epinephrine) is taken.
- Monitor BP and pulse at outset and every time blood taken.
- Take 2 baseline samples at 5-min intervals for catecholamines.
- At time 0, give 2.5mg pentolinium IV.
- Take blood at 10 and 20min.
- After 2h, measure BP and heart rate, supine and standing.
- Encourage patient to 'march on the spot' while standing in order to reduce venous pooling in the legs.
- If/when there is no symptomatic postural hypotension, the patient may now go home.

A positive result is 1 in which there is little or no fall in catecholamines (up to 8%) post-pentolinium, suggesting the presence of a phaeochromocytoma. Most normal patients should suppress between 22–63%.[1]

► Caution: after this test the patient should not drive for at least 6h and preferably not until the following day.

The benefit of this test is that pentolinium is short acting therefore any postural hypotension would be shortlived (up to 2h). However, it is renally excreted therefore should be used in patients with normal renal function. It also does not suppress NE levels much if the baseline level is normal.

This test is, generally, not used widely now.

Reference

1. Brown MJ, *et al.* (1981). Increased sensitivity and accuracy of phaeochromcytoma diagnosis achieved by use of plasma-adrenaline estimations and pentolinium suppression test. *Lancet* **1**:174–7.

Fludrocortisone suppression test

This is a test previously used to confirm the diagnosis of hyperaldosteronism. This is usually for patients with a suspected diagnosis of Conn's with either a low renin or an elevated aldosterone:renin ratio. The patient is admitted for 4 days to be given fludrocortisone orally, correcting for K^+. A baseline plasma and 24-h urinary aldosterone is measured prior to therapy. All diuretic therapies should have been omitted in the preceding 3 weeks.

Fludrocortisone (0.1mg) is given 6-hourly with sodium chloride 3 × a day (1.8g slow Na = 30mmol Na^+). A failure to suppress plasma aldosterone to <166pmol/L (assuming they are potassium replete—if not, they require supplementation) suggests 1° hyperaldosteronism. This is considered the gold standard test. It is contraindicated in patients with accelerated hypertension or heart failure.

Saline suppression test

- This can be used to confirm the diagnosis of hyperaldosteronism during a 1-day admission.
- 2L of saline 0.9% is administered over 4h as an infusion. Basal aldosterone and plasma renin activity is measured and rechecked at hourly intervals.
- The normal response is to suppress aldosterone <135pmol/L; if the aldosterone is between 135–270pmol/L, the result is thought to be borderline. A true case of 1° hyperaldosteronism would have values >270pmol/L.
- Both the fludrocortisone suppression test and saline suppression tests are not performed widely nowadays as current imaging techniques far exceed what was previously available, and inpatient stays for investigations are no longer practical nor cost effective.

Computed tomography

Computed tomography (CT) is generally reserved for patients in whom a 2° cause of hypertension is suspected.

Cardiac CT (electron beam/ultrafast CT) has the advantage of capturing images quickly and these are gated to the patient's ECG allowing the estimation of various functional parameters throughout the cardiac cycle. Calcium quantification (📖 Fig. 3.3) has been proposed as a potential screening tool for coronary artery disease—but the correlation between calcium and active inflamed plaque is unresolved—hence the absence of calcium does not exclude coronary disease.

Due to its radiation risks, the indication for requesting a CT has to be robust—this may include clinical signs and symptoms or biochemical evidence of underlying conditions. A CT chest may be useful to delineate the presence or absence of a coarctation of aorta and its position. A CT abdomen may help in the identification of an adrenal mass, e.g. phaeochromocytomas and paraganglionomas—and can help in the detection of adrenal adenomas—although frequently these are picked up as incidentalomas on scans performed for other indications. A CT may also delineate the anatomy of renal vessels when a RAS is suspected. Additionally, renal masses arising from polycystic kidneys, hypernephromas, or other conditions may be readily identified.

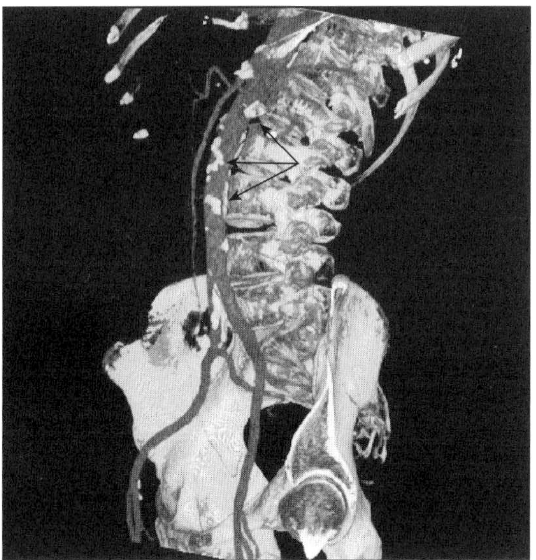

Fig. 3.3 3D volume rendered reconstruction on CT showing aortic calcification of the abdominal aorta (see arrows) (📖 see also Colour plate 9).

Magnetic resonance imaging

MRI is a useful, new, non-radioactive modality for imaging in 2° hypertension. It may be indicated in the investigation of adrenal hypertension, e.g. Conn's adenoma and RAS, and has the advantage over CT in terms of the lack of radiation.

Cardiac MRI allows excellent views of the anatomical structure of the heart and other great vessels of the CV tree. It has gained wide application in the diagnosis and treatment of congenital heart disease, coarctation, and dissection. Cine modalities have allowed the estimation of ejection fraction, anatomical dimensions, LVH, and mass estimations which are more reproducible than those obtainable by echocardiography. It is therefore useful when monitoring progress to therapy in research studies but its limitations are availability and expertise (as well as prolonged imaging time)—which, currently, is still limited to large teaching hospitals.

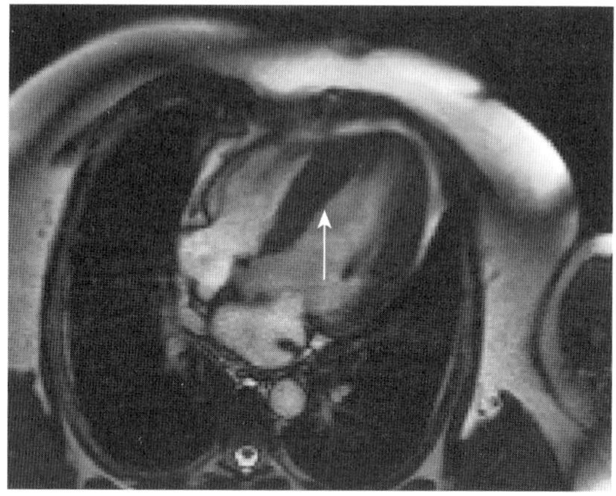

Fig. 3.4 MRI showing LVH (arrow) (courtesy of Dr JHF Rudd, Cambridge).

Nuclear medicine: adrenal

Nuclear medicine can provide some clues as to the underlying causes of 2° hypertension—which may be requested based on the history or once biochemistry provides a clue. The type of nuclear medicine scan depends on the diagnosis being queried.

MIBG scan

MIBG scintigraphy is useful in the anatomical localization of phaeochromocytomas especially once the biochemical diagnosis has been made on urinary metanephrines (or VMA) or plasma catecholamines and CT scanning or MRI has revealed the presence of a mass.

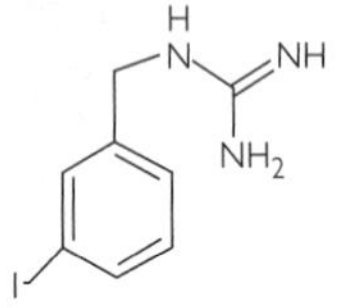

Fig. 3.5 Chemical structure of MIBG.

MIBG has a structure similar to NE (Fig. 3.5) and is taken up by neuroendocrine tumours such as phaeochromocytomas (see Fig. 3.6) but also paraganglionomas, neuroblastomas, carcinoid, and medullary thyroid carcinomas). It is usually labelled with ^{123}I or ^{131}I—the former is usually used for diagnosis and the latter for therapeutic use—although this is not exclusively so.

Drugs which interfere with the scan should be stopped (including antipsychotics, antihypertensives, opioids, tricyclics, and sympathomimetics) prior to the scan. Iodine is given orally for a few days prior to injection of MIBG to block uptake in the thyroid gland. A 5-min image is taken and a repeat whole body scan is done within 18–24h. Whilst MIBG also accumulates physiologically in certain organs, abnormal uptake in areas correlating to abnormal masses on other imaging modalities helps to confirm the diagnosis. More recently, MIBG-SPECT can be combined with images on CT or MRI allowing for co-registration of the functional and anatomical components (see Fig. 3.7).

Once the diagnosis is established, MIBG uptake means that chemical treatment can be deployed using higher doses of radiolabelled ^{131}I-MIBG to treat the tumour and monitor its progress thereafter using ^{123}I-MIBG. It is usually used in inoperable cases where the tumour shows uptake in all metastatic sites. A negative MIBG scan (which can occur in 15% of benign and 50% of malignant phaeochromocytoma) usually means therapeutic intervention using MIBG will not be possible. The usual reasons for MIBG negative phaeochromocytomas include small tumour size, central necrosis, or haemorrhage and tumour location. MIBG should not be used as a therapeutic modality for small intra-adrenal phaeochromocytomas.

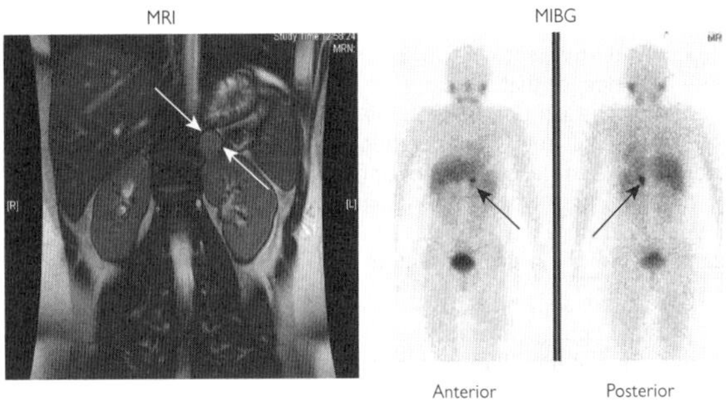

Fig. 3.6 MRI (left) showing a left-sided adrenal mass (see arrow). This was then confirmed on MIBG scan (arrowed on anterior and posterior views) to be a phaeochromocytoma. Note also the physiological uptake in the liver, salivary glands, and bladder.

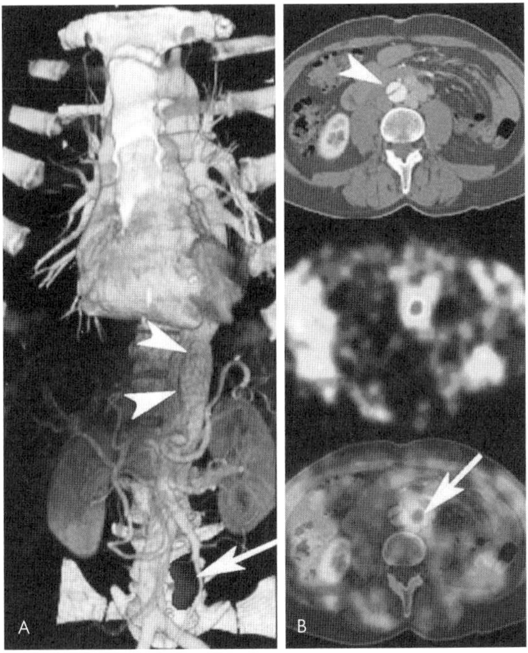

Fig. 3.7 MIBG-SPECT combined with CT showing a paraganglionoma with MIBG uptake (arrow) and a Type B dissection of the aorta (arrowheads) in the same patient. Reproduced from Strobel K, *et al.* (2007). MIBG-SPECT/CT-angiography with 3-D reconstruction of an extra-adrenal phaeochromocytoma with dissection of an aortic aneurysm *Eur J Nuc Med Mol Imaging* **34**:150, with permission (📖 also see Colour plate 11).

PET-CT scans

MIBG scans may sometimes be negative for phaeochromocytomas. There is ↑ evidence that functional imaging using PET-CT scans (📖 Fig. 3.8) may localize the anatomical locations of phaeochromocytomas more accurately in these patients. Consideration should be given to functional imaging if there is biochemical evidence of a phaeochromocytoma but initial imaging with MIBG is negative. Functional imaging itself may be specific or non-specific—therefore if a specific test is negative, then a more non-specific test may reveal the malignant tumour, especially if metastatic (📖 Fig. 3.9).

^{18}F-FDA (fluorodopamine) has been shown to be superior to ^{131}I-MIBG in metastatic phaeochromocytoma—including those which are MIBG negative. ^{18}F-FDOPA (fluorodihydroxyphenylalanine) has 100% sensitivity and specificity. ^{18}F-FDG is less sensitive as it is non-specifically taken up by metabolically active tissue.

In VHL, underexpression of NE transporter in VHL-related phaeochromocytomas may explain low sensitivity 97%) with MIBG—where ^{18}F-FDA has a sensitivity of 100%.[2] This may be important when screening for VHL.

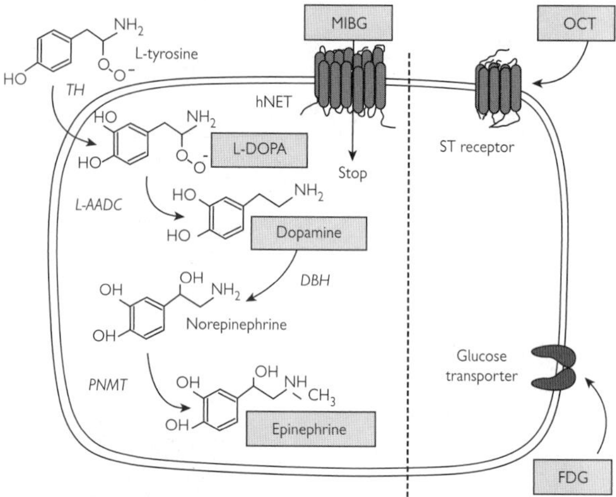

Fig. 3.8 Potential functional imaging targets within the chromaffin cell. Specific targets are on the left, less specific on the right. The boxed substances can be radiolabelled for use in PET-CT. hNET, human norepinephrine transporter; ST, somatostatin Adapted from Ilias I, *et al.* (2005). New functional imaging modalities for chromaffin tumors, neuroblastomas and ganglioneuromas. *Trends Endocrinol Metab* **16**:66–72, © 2005, with permission from Elsevier.

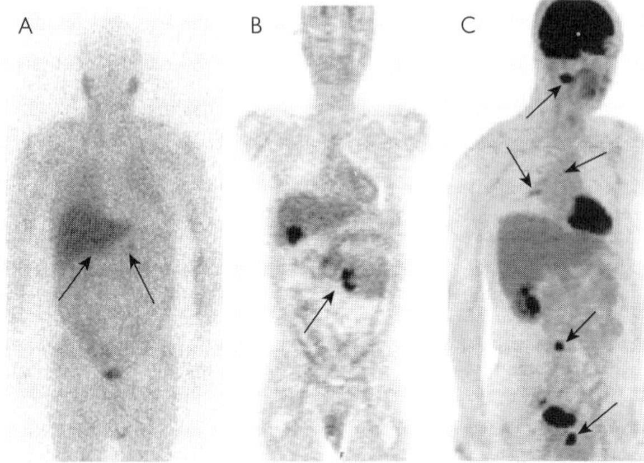

Fig. 3.9 (A) ^{123}I-MIBG shows adrenal uptake (arrows). (B) ^{18}F-FDOPA-PET shows left paranephric extra-adrenal phaeochromocytoma (arrow). (C) ^{18}FDG-PET shows spinal, pelvic, and rib metastases (arrowed). Reproduced from Mackenzie IS, *et al.* (2007). *Eur J Endocrinol* **157**:533–7. © 2007 Society of the European Journal of Endocrinology, with permission.

References

1. Ilias I, *et al.* (2005). New functional imaging modalities for chromaffin tumors, neuroblastomas and ganglioneuromas. *Trends Endocrinol Metab* **16**:66–72.
2. Kaji P, *et al.* (2007). The role of 6-[18F]fluorodopamine positron emission tomography in the localization of adrenal pheochromocytoma associated with von Hippel–Lindau syndrome. *Eur J Endocrinol* **156**: 483–7.

Nuclear medicine: kidney

Isotope renography provides functional and anatomical information about kidneys which may help in the diagnosis of kidney disorders in general and occasionally underlying causes of hypertension—in particular RAS.

A variety of isotopes can be used including DTPA and MAG-3.

MAG 3 renogram scan

MAG-3 renal scintigrams offer information about kidney structure and function. It provides physiologic information to complement information gathered from other imaging modalities. It effectively provides a gauge of effective renal plasma flow as most of it is excreted via tubular secretion in the proximal tubule via an active transporter. Therefore, MAG 3 extraction is reduced in patients with impaired renal function. There are also pitfalls when investigating patients with bilateral stenoses and those on concurrent antihypertensives.

MAG 3 renograms are normally performed with and without an ACEI challenge—which essentially determines the functionality of the stenosis which may have been diagnosed using another modality. An ACEI also dramatically ↑ the sensitivity and specificity of the test—so the ACEI challenge is usually performed before the unchallenged scan. The second scan is only done if the ACEI challenge is positive. A positive MAG 3 with captopril study is also said to predict a hypertensive cure or improvement following vascular intervention, whereas a stenotic lesion with no change suggests poor surgical curability.

MAG 3 has a sensitivity and specificity of around 90% in centres that perform them frequently but they are less predictive than MR angiography which has obvious advantages especially in patients with impaired renal function.

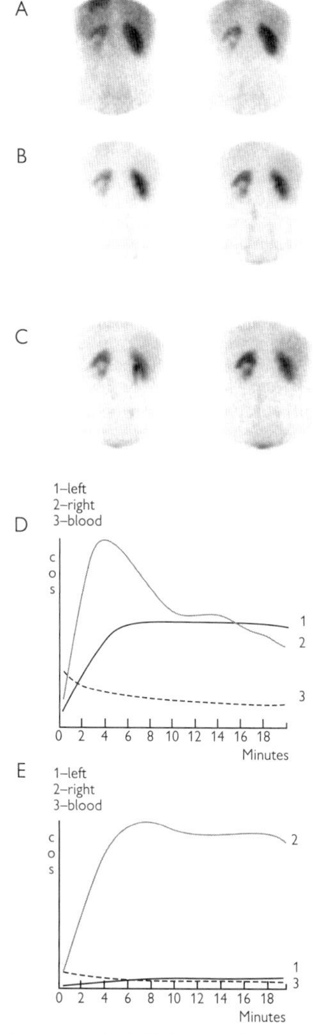

Fig. 3.10 MAG-3 scintigram result (A–C) showing a functional RAS of the left renal artery. (A) and (B) show reduced tracer uptake for the left kidney. The excretion graphs (D) and (E) show flat uptake and release of tracer suggesting a left RAS. (D) is pre-captopril challenge; (E) is post-captopril challenge.

Interventional radiology

In a few select patients, interventional radiological techniques may help establish the diagnosis.

Renal arteriograms were routinely performed in the past to diagnose RAS. With the advent of superior imaging modalities such as CT and MRI, this has now been superseded. Nevertheless, it remains the gold standard investigation for RAS with a 100% sensitivity and specificity for the diagnosis. There is still a role for invasive angiography if a decision is made to either measure the gradient across the lesion, obtain samples for renin (renal vein renin sampling), or to perform angioplasty to the previously identified lesion.

Adrenal vein sampling (AVS) is a technique to determine whether the biochemically determined syndrome of hyperaldosteronism is unilateral or bilateral and if an apparent adenoma on CT is indeed a functioning adenoma. Excision of unilateral adenomas may result in amelioration, if not cure, of hypertension. It may, rarely, also be performed in adrenal Cushing's disease or in bilateral adrenal hyperplasia.

The technique requires cannulation of the femoral vein and the passage of a guidewire for sampling of both adrenal veins—something requiring the skills of an experienced interventional radiologist. A common pitfall is failure to cannulate the adrenal vein itself, especially on the right side, as it is smaller and comes off the inferior vena cava itself.

Cortisol levels from the adrenal veins should be twice as high as those obtained from the inferior vena cava. If this is not the case, the sampling should not be interpreted. An aldosterone/cortisol gradient of ≥2 (compared to contralateral adrenal vein) is considered diagnostic of an adrenal adenoma if the non-affected side is higher than the gradient measured in the inferior vena cava. Bilateral adrenal hyperplasia tends to cause gradients higher than peripheral samples. Complications include adrenal infarction, thrombosis, haemorrhage, hypotension, and adrenal insufficiency. Other pitfalls include concomitant medications which may skew the results of sampling; hence the omission of aldosterone antagonists, in particular, is vital.

There was a vogue for performing adrenocorticotrophic hormone (ACTH) stimulation during AVS, but this has been abandoned to some extent, as it may make interpretation of the results more difficult.

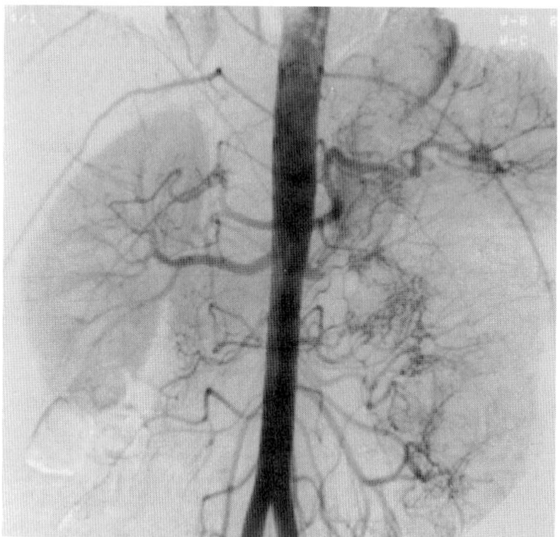

Fig. 3.11 A renal arteriogram performed to diagnose a left RAS.

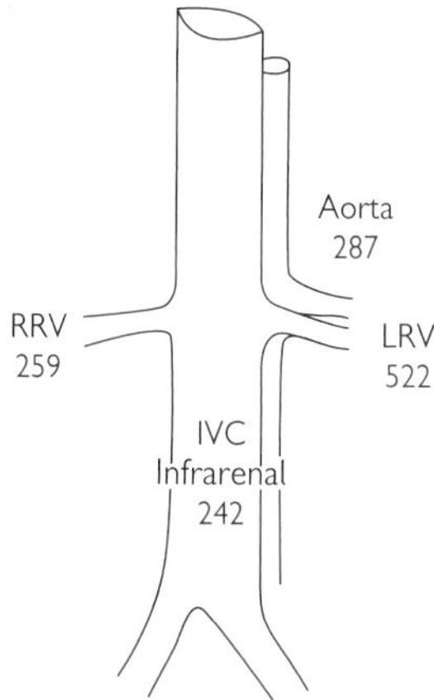

Renin levels (in mU/L), normal random renin range 9–56 mU/L

Fig. 3.12 A pictorial representation of the same patient in Fig 3.11 showing results of renal vein renin sampling. This shows lateralization to the left renal vein indicating a higher production of renin from that side—implicating that kidney as the cause of hypertension in this patient. IVC, inferior vena cava; LRV, left renal vein; RRV, right renal vein.

Chapter 4

Secondary hypertension

Co-arctation of the aorta

Background

Co-arctation refers to a congenital narrowing of the aorta, due to localized thickening of the media, the exact pathophysiology of which is unknown. The lesion usually occurs just distal to the origin of the left subclavian artery (distal to the ductus arteriosus), but rarely may be in the latter part of the descending thoracic or abdominal aorta. The degree of narrowing may vary from a distinct tight band to a more extensive lesion involving a segment of aorta. Co-arctation results in upper body hypertension, probably due to impaired renal artery perfusion, and consequent activation of the RAAS.

Demographics

The prevalence of co-arctation is ~1/10,000 with a male:female ratio of 2:1. Co-arctation is usually diagnosed in childhood, presenting as hypertension or cardiac failure. However, a significant proportion remains undetected until adolescence or early adulthood, and is often picked up as 'essential' hypertension or 'incidental' murmurs. Occasionally, co-arctation may present as malignant hypertension.

Co-arctation accounts for ~5% of cases of congenital heart disease, and is often associated with other cardiac abnormalities, including bicuspid aortic valve (~50% of cases), ventricular-septal defect, and aortic stenosis. Up to 10% of patients may also have associated cerebral aneurysms which may be multiple. Co-arctation is also a recognized feature of Turner's syndrome.

Clinical features

- Upper body hypertension with a difference of at least 10mmHg in systolic pressure between the arms and the legs.
- Diminished or delayed femoral pulses (radio-femoral delay).
- A systolic murmur heard over the back (which may be continuous if the co-arctation is severe). An associated aortic systolic murmur may be present if there is a bicuspid aortic valve.
- A forceful apex beat (due to LVH).

Investigations

Routine blood tests are usually normal, although renin levels may be raised in some individuals. The ECG typically shows LVH, and CXR may show the classical features of a dilated ascending aorta and rib notching caused by collateral vessels eroding the ribs. Transthoracic echocardiography may not reveal the co-arctation itself, but frequently reveals LVH or a bicuspid aortic valve.

The definitive investigation is CT or MR angiography, which will not only confirm the diagnosis but reveal the site and severity of the lesion (📖 Fig. 4.1). Conventional angiography is now rarely performed except in more complex cases or as a prelude to non-surgical intervention.

Management

If left untreated, 20% of patients with co-arctation die before the age of 20 years, and 80% before age 50. Classically, the definitive treatment has been surgical correction, which has the best outcome if performed in childhood between the ages of 1–7 years. If correction is not performed until later, long-term hypertension is more likely. Post-operatively there is occasionally a marked rise in BP which is thought to be due to disruption of the baro-reflex arc, and may be prevented by preoperative β-blockade.

Recently there has been a trend away from surgery and towards balloon angioplasty (with or without stent insertion). Although widely accepted, and high technical success rates have been reported, only limited long-term follow-up data are available, and there are few head-to-head comparisons with surgical intervention. Angioplasty may also be associated with an ↑ risk of aneurysm formation and re-stenosis. Nevertheless, in children and young adults with uncomplicated lesions, many cardiologists opt for angioplasty 1st-line.

Despite good haemodynamic responses to intervention, ~20% of patients will remain hypertensive, probably due to permanent structural changes in the CV system and neurohormonal adaptation. Recurrence of the lesion may also occur in ~10% of cases operated on in childhood, and possibly a higher number post-angioplasty.

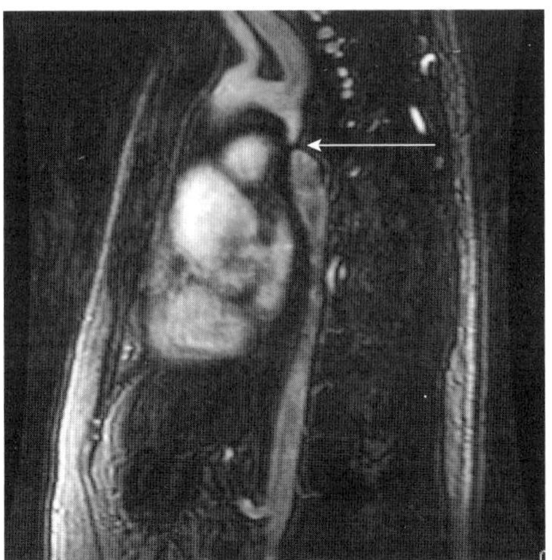

Fig. 4.1 Cardiac MRI of a 22-year-old with co-arctation distal to the left subclavian artery (arrow). Note the dilatation of the inominate and subclavian arteries.

Renal artery stenosis

Background

RAS refers to a narrowing of the renal arteries, which may or may not be causally linked with hypertension, renal impairment, or 'flash' pulmonary oedema. Indeed, there is a complex relationship between these 3 clinical presentations, and in some cases the stenosis may simply be an innocent bystander (📖 Fig. 4.2). Reno-vascular hypertension refers to the situation where RAS leads to the development of 2° hypertension.

The mechanism of hypertension in RAS is complex and depends on whether one or both kidneys are involved. In classical, unilateral RAS, the initial elevation of BP is due to reduced renal blood flow, and activation of the renin–angiotensin system. Although renin levels may fall somewhat, this mechanism remains important in the longer term but is augmented by structural changes in the contralateral kidney which, together with higher circulating levels of aldosterone, limit its ability to excrete sodium, and hence there is an expansion of plasma volume. In bilateral RAS the initial phase of hypertension is similar but volume expansion is much more important in the chronic phase and renin levels are often normal or only marginally raised.

Demographics

The true prevalence of reno-vascular hypertension is unknown, not least because of the difficulty in establishing causality. However, estimates range from <1% in unselected populations to 30% amongst subjects with resistant hypertension in 2° care.

Causes of RAS

- Atherosclerotic disease: 85%.
- Fibromuscular dysplasia: 10%.
- Others, 5%:
  - Dissecting aneurysm.
  - Trauma.
  - Embolism/thrombosis.
  - Neurofibromatosis.
  - Radiation fibrosis.
  - Arteritis.

Atherosclerotic RAS

Classically, affects older individuals, especially male cigarette smokers. Individuals frequently have widespread atherosclerosis and concomitant peripheral vascular and coronary disease, and it is probably under-diagnosed (12% of patients undergoing coronary angiography have significant RAS). It usually primarily affects the proximal 1/3 of the main renal artery, and tends to be progressive. Total occlusion may occur, and is estimated at between 30–60% at 4–7 years. Renal atrophy develops in ~20% of individuals with a stenosis >60%. Besides hypertension, atherosclerotic RAs may present with a sudden deterioration in renal function or BP, or rarely 'flash pulmonary oedema' if bilateral.

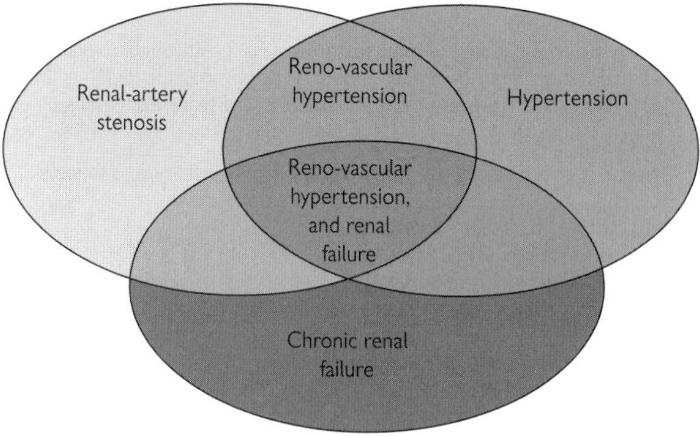

Fig. 4.2 Overlap between RAS, hypertension, and renal failure.

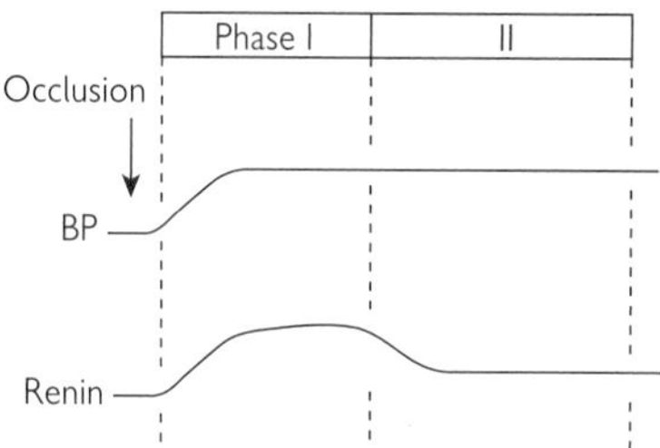

Fig. 4.3 Physiology of unilateral RAS.

Fibromuscular dysplasia (FMD)

Typically affects young females (4:1). Although most cases are sporadic, some have a familial tendency, which tend to display a dominant pattern of inheritance with incomplete penetrance. Any layer of the arterial wall may be affected, but most commonly the media. The underlying pathology remains unclear but may involve ischemia of the vasa vasorum. Histologically, FMD is characterized by fibrotic stenosis and aneurysmal dilatation which gives rise to the classical string of beads appearance at angiography (📖 Fig. 4.4). Frequently involves the distal 2/3 of the renal artery and their branches, and ~40% of cases have bilateral involvement. Total occlusion and progression are uncommon (~1/3 of cases). Extra-renal arteries may be involved too, e.g. cerebral or carotid.

Clinical features

There are no true pathognomonic features of RAS. Although a 'renal' bruit is classically described, in reality this is of poor prognostic value. Many patients have clinical evidence of atherosclerotic disease elsewhere.

Features suggestive of RAS

- Onset of hypertension <30 years with no family history or other risk factors.
- Refractory or resistant hypertension.
- Malignant hypertension.
- Known PVD or aortic aneurysm.
- Worsening renal function (particularly after introduction of ACEI).
- Renal atrophy.
- Flash pulmonary oedema (bilateral disease).
- Abdominal (renal) bruit.

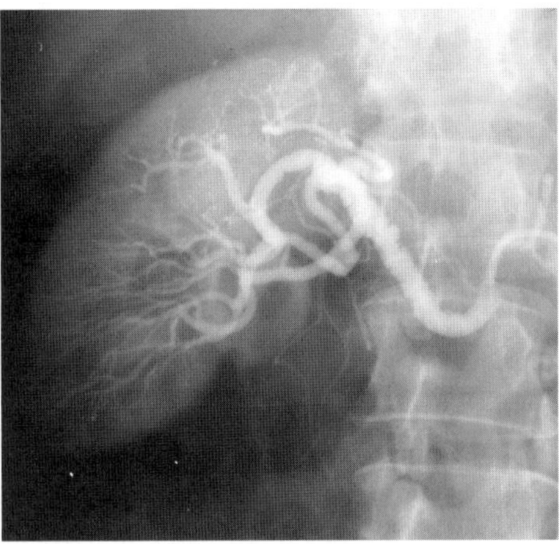

Fig. 4.4 Typical 'string-of-beads' or 'corkscrew' appearance of FMD in a 27-year-old woman.

Investigations

Basic blood tests should be performed, together with urine analysis and an ECG. Inflammatory markers and autoantibodies should be considered if a vasculitic process is suspected. Investigating suspected RAS is a 2-step process: 1st screen for the condition and, if positive, 2nd confirm the diagnosis and assess severity. MR-angiography is increasingly used to do both at a single setting, especially when clinical suspicion is high, although cost and availability limit its total adoption. An ideal 3rd step would be to assess the physiological severity and likely impact of corrective therapy, but as yet there is no suitable test.

Screening tests

- Renin and aldosterone (📖 see Renin and aldosterone, p.72). May be helpful—classically both should be raised, but a 'normal' plasma renin does not usefully exclude the diagnosis. Assessing the response to a single dose of captopril has been suggested, but this has poor sensitivity and specificity for detecting RAS.
- Renal ultrasound. Helps exclude obstruction if there is renal impairment and to assess kidney size. Unequal size or bilaterally small kidney may be a helpful pointer to RAS.
- Renal artery Doppler. Stenotic lesions are detected by examining the flow velocity profile, and comparing velocities of the renal artery to the aorta. In subjects with a high pre-test probability for RAS the sensitivity and specificity are high, ~98%, but much less lower if the pre-test probability is low. Overall the technique is very operator- (and patient-) dependent.
- Captopril renography (📖 see MAG 3, p.130). DTPA or MAG 3 isotope scans are widely available but have a poor performance if used alone. The sensitivity and specificity is dramatically improved when combined with captopril administration (>90%). However, there is no direct imaging of the renal vessels, and predictive value falls in subjects on anti-hypertensive medication and if there is significant renal impairment.
- CT-angiography (📖 see p.123). Provides 3D images of the renal arteries and aorta (📖 Fig. 4.5). Has a sensitivity of 98% and specificity of 94% compared with invasive angiography, but a variable sensitivity in FMD. Unfortunately, it involves potentially nephrotoxic contrast medium, ionizing radiation
- MR-angiography (📖 see p.124). Increasingly used as 1st-line screening test. Provides 3D images of the renal arteries and aorta, but distal lesions are more difficult to detect. Two small studies showed a sensitivity of 100% and specificity of 71–96% when compared to arteriography. Less useful for diagnosis of FMD. There have also been recent concerns about the long-term safety of gadolinium contrast agents in patients with renal failure.

Confirmatory tests

The 'gold-standard' test remains invasive angiography, which has the advantage that pressure gradients can also be assessed and intervention performed at the same time in suitable patients. However, it is associated with the use of ionizing radiation, and a small but significant risk of complications, e.g. dissection and haemorrhage. Therefore, CT or MRI may be used in some setting to confirm the diagnosis.

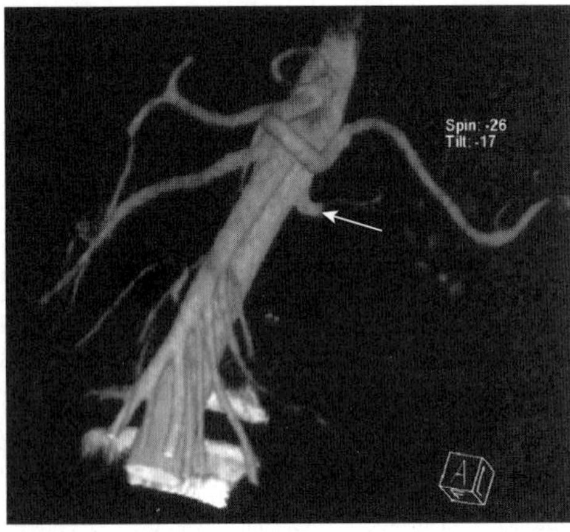

Fig. 4.5 CT-angiogram illustrating complete occlusion of the left renal artery (arrow).

Treatment

The key aims of therapy are to control BP, preserve or improve renal function, and stabilize the lesion. The decision to opt for medical therapy or revascularization will depend on a number of factors including the nature of the lesion, patient's age, and co-morbidity, and requires careful consideration. Overall, it should be noted that only a few patients with reno-vascular hypertension are truly cured by intervention.

Medical therapy

ACEI and ARAs are effective in controlling BP in the majority of individuals, especially when combined with a diuretic. However, they should not be used if there is bilateral disease, and U&Es should be closely monitored, as acute renal insufficiency can occur even in unilateral disease (5–10% of cases). A rise in the serum creatinine >25% should lead to withdrawal of the agent. CCAs may also be helpful, and are less likely to induce renal failure. There is little hard evidence that adequate BP control preserves renal function. Moreover, a significant number of subjects will fail to achieve targets despite multiple drug therapy. Statin therapy is also widely used in subjects with atherosclerotic RAS. However, only 1 small study suggests a reduction in rate progression of the stenotic lesion, and there seems no effect on renal function[1].

Revascularization

In general, the results of surgical intervention and angioplasty have been disappointing. Although good technical results can be obtained in the majority of patients, long-term 'cure' rates are low, and the effect on renal function very modest. This must be balanced against the perceived risks of lesion progression and also the risks of intervention (~3% risk of serious complications).

In general, the best results are seen in younger subjects, those with FMD, or recent onset disease. Significant renal impairment, small kidneys, and advanced age are all associated with a worse outcome. Occasionally, revascularization may be undertaken in subjects with refractory heart failure and RAS. Although renal vein renin and the response to ACEI have been suggested as predictors of the response to revascularization, in general these are unreliable.

Angioplasty

Angioplasty, increasingly with stent insertion, is the most common form of revascularization. Although good technical results are common, the evidence base is very modest, and in atherosclerotic RAS the results have been generally very disappointing. The DRASTIC study is the largest RCT undertaken in this setting, and compared angioplasty with medical therapy in 106 patients with uncontrolled hypertension. There was no difference in BP, or the use of antihypertensives, or renal function after 12 months' follow-up. The ASTRAL and CORAL studies are ongoing and will address the use of stents and angioplasty in a larger cohort. In subjects with FMD, the results are considerably better: ~50% of patients are cured, and the majority have better BP control.

Surgery

The results are very similar to angioplasty. However, surgery may be a better option if there is extrinsic compression, or a difficult ostial stenosis. Again better results are likely in younger subjects with recent onset disease. Occasionally, unilateral nephrectomy is performed to remove a non-functioning kidney thought to be driving hypertension through renin release.

Reference

1. Cheung CM, *et al.* (2007). The effects of statins on the progression of atherosclerotic renovascular disease. *Nephron Clin Pract* **107**:c35–c42.

Hyperaldosteronism

Production of the mineralocorticoid aldosterone by the zona glomerulosa is usually closely regulated by angiotensin II and serum potassium levels, and thus depends on intravascular volume and body sodium. Hyperaldosteronism refers to excess production of aldosterone by the adrenal gland, and is traditionally sub-divided into 1° and 2° hyperaldosteronism based on the plasma renin. It is the 2nd most common form of 2° hypertension after renal disorders.

1° hyperaldosteronism

The excess production of aldosterone originates from within the adrenal gland itself, and is not regulated by the normal feedback mechanisms. As such, plasma renin is suppressed, i.e. low (mass <5mU/L; activity <0.65ng/mL/h). This is usually accompanied by hypokalaemia, alkalosis, and sometimes mild hypernatraemia. However, it is important to note that the plasma K^+ is normal in a substantial proportion of patients with 1° hyperaldosteronism, and may only fall with diuretic therapy. Clinically, the hypokalaemia may rarely manifest as weakness, fatigue, paraesthesia, and cramps. Hypertension is common and results from sodium and water retention, and a consequent expansion in plasma volume, but CNS effects including sympathetic activation and enhanced sodium intake are also important.

The true incidence of 1° hyperaldosteronism is difficult to establish, not least because of widely varying diagnostic criteria. Although once considered rare, most current estimates suggest an incidence amongst hypertensive subjects of ~5–10%. It is more common in subjects with resistant hypertension, and obviously those with appropriate electrolyte abnormalities.

Causes

- Adrenal adenoma (Conn's syndrome): ~70%.
- Bilateral adrenal hyperplasia: ~25%.
- Adrenal adenocarcinoma: rare.
- Glucocorticoid-remediable hyperaldosteronism (📖 see Glucocorticoid remediable aldosteronism, p.178): very rare.

Investigations

Anyone suspected of 1° hyperaldosteronism, e.g. appropriate electrolyte abnormalities, resistant hypertension, or an adrenal mass, should undergo biochemical screening.

Screening

The key screening test is the aldosterone:renin ratio (ARR), (📖 see Renin and aldosterone, p.72). Table 4.1 provides a guide for cut-off values for diagnosing 1° hyperaldosteronism, with ~95% sensitivity and a ~75% specificity.

Table 4.1 Cut-off levels for the ARR, above which a diagnosis of 1° hyperaldosteronism is likely

	Renin activity		Renin mass	
Aldosterone	**ng/mL/h**	**pmol/L/min**	**μU/mL**	**ng/L**
ng/dL	27	2.1	3.3	5.4
pmol/L	750	59	90	150

Adapted from Sealey JE, *et al.* (2005). Plasma renin and aldosterone measurements in low renin hypertensive states. *Trends Endocrinol Metab* **16**:86–91 © 2005, with permission from Elsevier.

It is important to appreciate that the test is unreliable if the aldosterone levels are low as a low renin level can still produce a positive result. Therefore, most centres have an arbitrary level of aldosterone, e.g. 300pmol/L, below which the ARR should not be calculated. Moreover, drug therapy, particularly β-blockade and spironolactone, may confound the results. If the ARR is suggestive of 1° hyperaldosteronism, then confirmatory tests should be performed. These can be thought of biochemical confirmation, and imaging to help confirm and localize any lesion.

Confirmatory tests

A number of confirmatory tests have been proposed including salt loading (🕮 see Salt suppression test, p.122), fludrocortisone suppression (🕮 see Fludrocortisone suppression test, p.122), infusion of angiotensin II, and selective venous sampling. Each has its own advantages and disadvantages, and the precise choice will depend heavily on local expertise. Although technically demanding and invasive, selective venous sampling probably remains the 'gold-standard' confirmatory test (🕮 see Interventional radiology, p.132). Generally, patients are withdrawn from mineralocorticoid antagonists and of potential confounding medications such as CCAs for up to 1 week before sampling. It is important to assess cortisol as well as aldosterone to ensure cannulation of the adrenal vein (the right is particularly difficult), and a positive result is generally considered to be a >3-fold difference between sides.

One schema is to perform either salt-loading or fludrocortisone suppression, and, then if positive, to perform selective venous sampling. If there is a high clinical suspicion and/or positive imaging then just undertaking venous sampling may be appropriate.

Imaging

Either high resolution CT or MRI (📖 Fig. 4.6) can be used to assess the adrenal glands. The choice depends on availability and local expertise. Imaging is useful in identifying potential adenomas (or carcinomas), or noting their absence, but interpretation is best in the context of the results of the confirmatory tests noted above. Isotope scanning is now rarely performed due to a lack of substrate, but newer PET ligands are in development.

Treatment

Treatment is discussed under the sub-types of 1° hyperaldosteronism that follow in this chapter.

2° hyperaldosteronism

Here the excess aldosterone production is driven through the normal regulatory pathways by factors extrinsic to the adrenal gland. This is usually, but not always, by an excess of plasma renin. Hypertension may or may not be present.

Causes

- Volume depletion.
- Cardiac failure.
- RAS.
- Malignant hypertension.
- Hepatic failure.

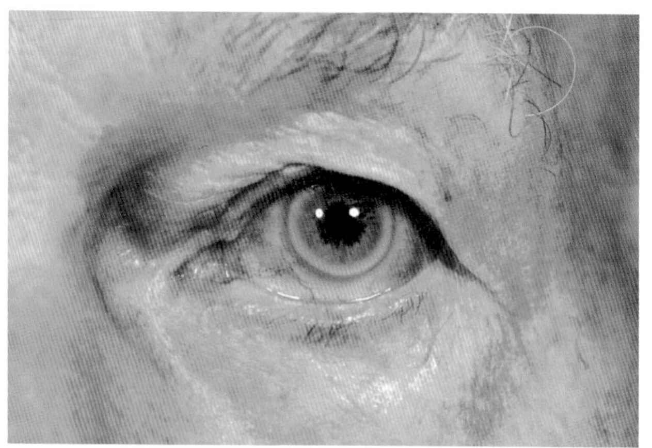

Colour plate 1 Corneal arcus (arcus senilis) (📖 see p.62)

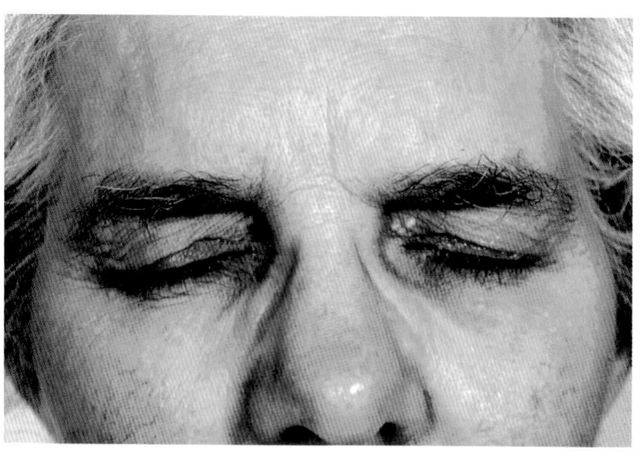

Colour plate 2 Xanthelasma (📖 see p.62)

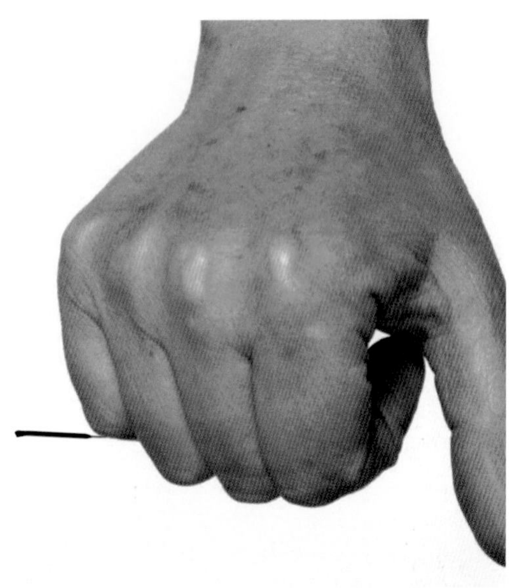

Colour plate 3 Tendon xanthomata (📖 see p.62)

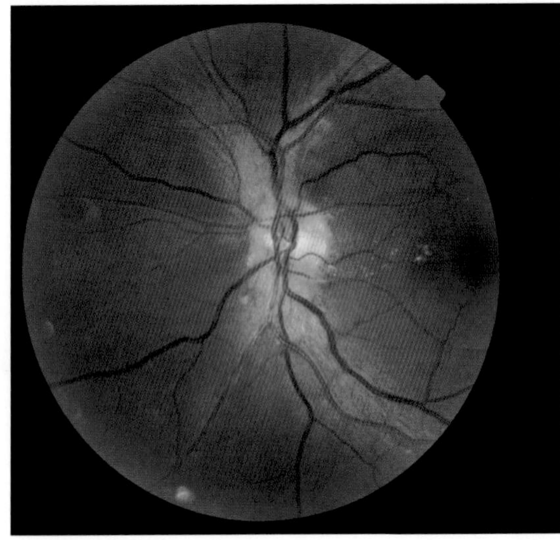

Colour plate 4 Grade 3 hypertensive retinopathy—silver wiring, AV nipping and soft exudates (📖 see also p.63)

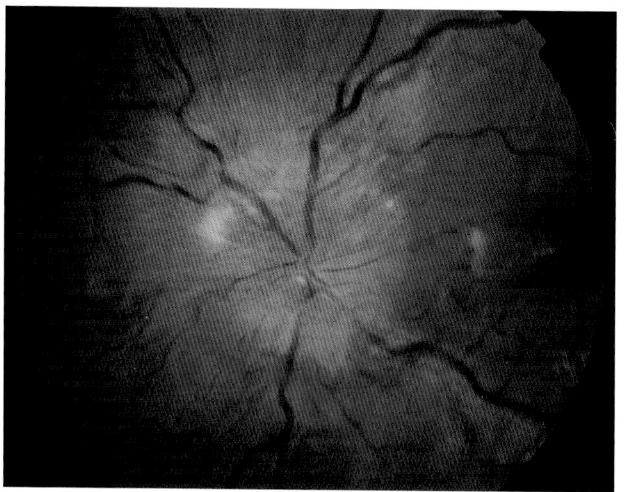

Colour plate 5 Grade IV hypertensive retinopathy with papilloedema (see also, Fig. 2.6, p.63)

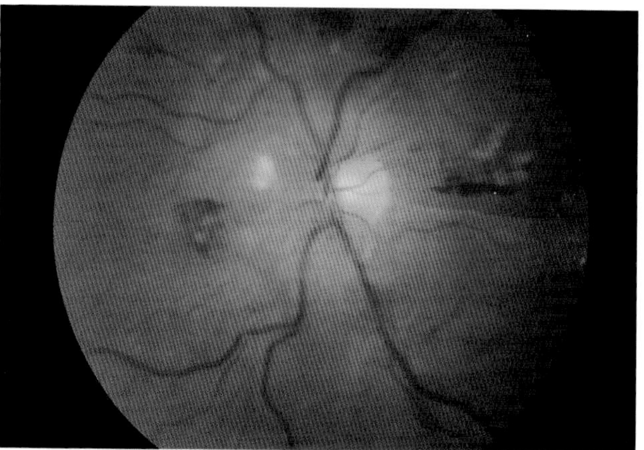

Colour plate 6 Grade IV hypertensive retinopathy with papilloedema, retinal haemorrhages, soft exudates/cotton wool spots and retinal oedema (see also, Fig. 2.6, p.63)

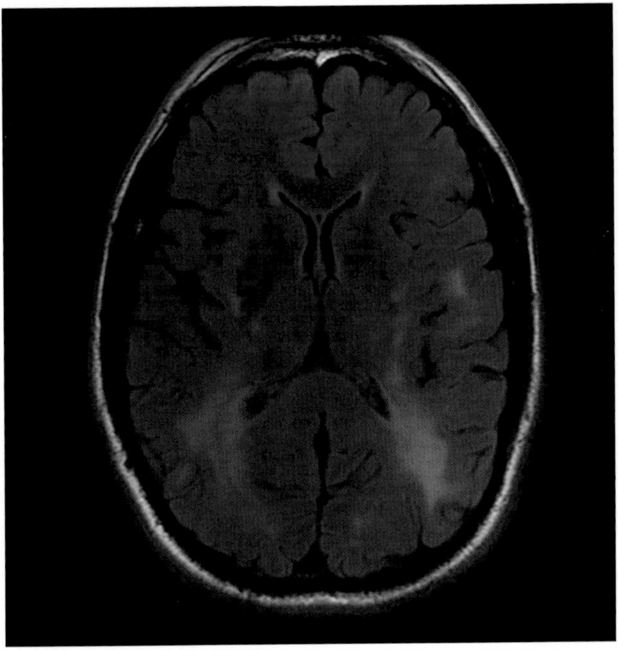

Colour plate 7 Posterior reversible leukoencephalopathy syndrome (PRES)—disordered cerebral autoregulation leading to vasogenic oedema presenting with altered mental state, headaches, seizures, and visual loss or other variable neurological abnormalities with classical radiological abnormalities—especially in the parieto-occipital regions. Severe uncontrolled hypertension or immunosuppression leading to endothelial dysfunction is implicated in the pathogenesis (📖 see p.109)

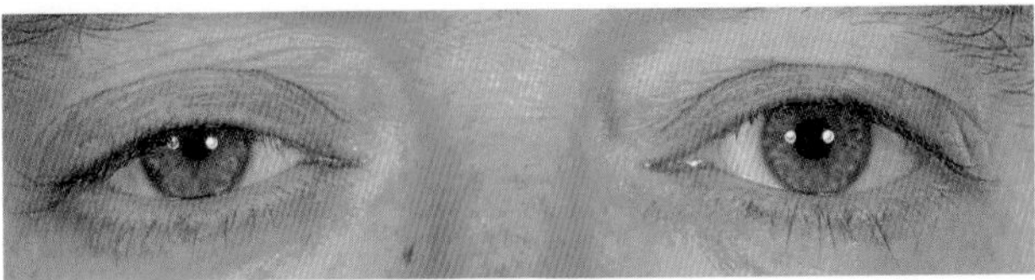

Colour plate 8 The same patient with PRES—who presented with a right sided Horner's syndrome (📖 see p.109)

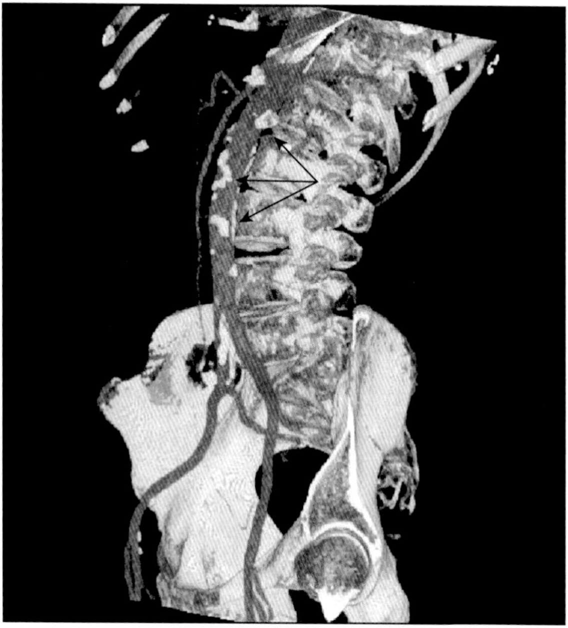

Colour plate 9 3D volume rendered CT reconstruction demonstrating aortic calcification of the abdominal aorta (see arrows) (📖 see Fig. 3.3, p.123)

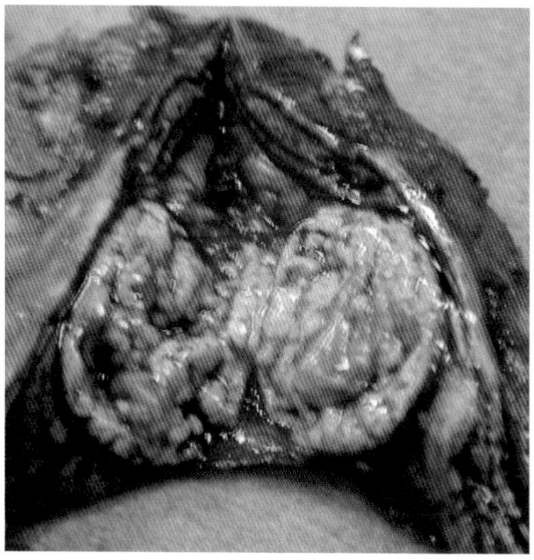

Colour plate 10 Example of a Conn's tumour (📖 see also Fig. 4.7, p.149)

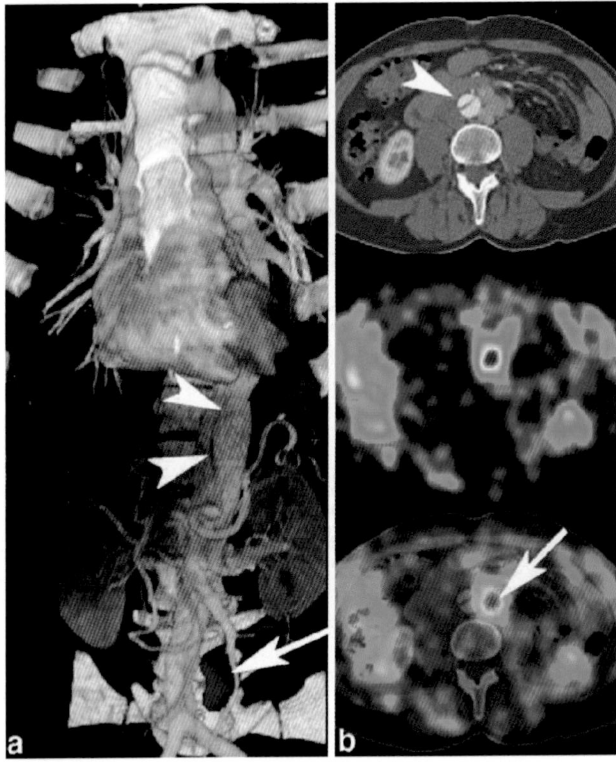

Colour plate 11 MIBG-SPECT combined with CT showing a paraganglionoma with MIBG uptake (arrow) and a Type B dissection of the aorta (arrowheads) in the same patient. Reproduced from Strobel K *et al.* (2007). MIBG-SPECT/CT-angiography with 3-D reconstruction of an extra-adrenal phaeochromocytoma with dissection of an aortic aneurysm. *Eur J Nuc Med Mol Imaging* **34**: 150, with permission (📖 see also Fig 3.7, p.127)

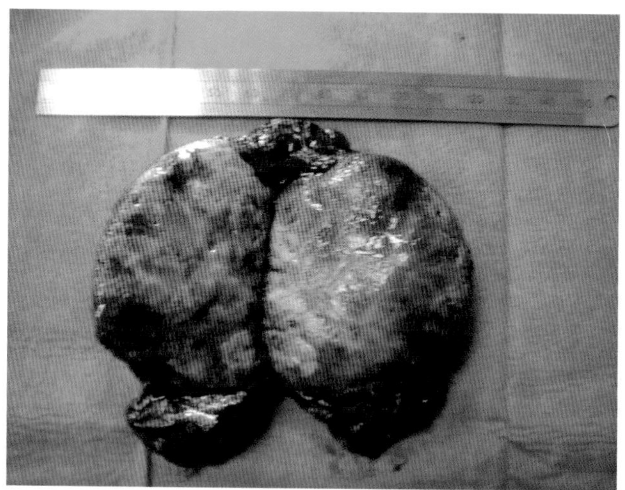

Colour plate 12 Example of a benign phaeochromocytoma (📖 see also Fig. 4.10, p.153)

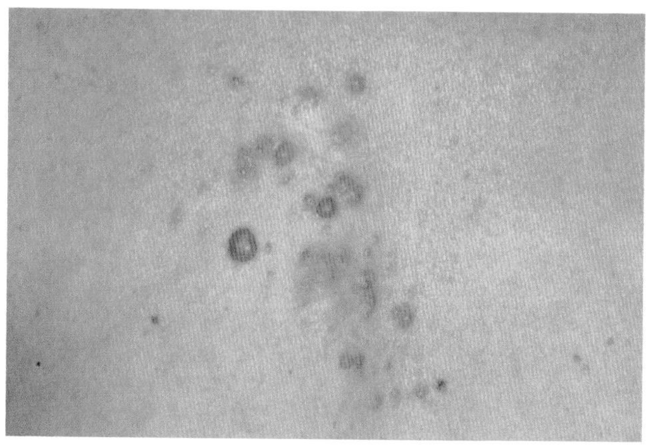

Colour plate 13 Neurofibromatosis—which can be associated with phaeochromocytoma (📖 see p.152)

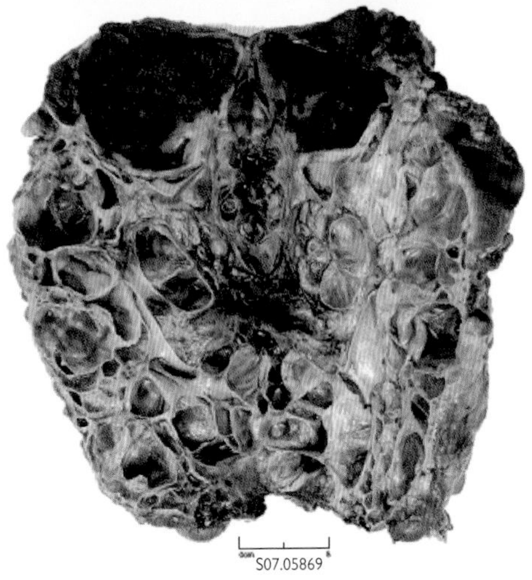

Colour plate 14 A microscopic view of a polycystic kidney
(📖 see also Fig. 4.13, p.161)

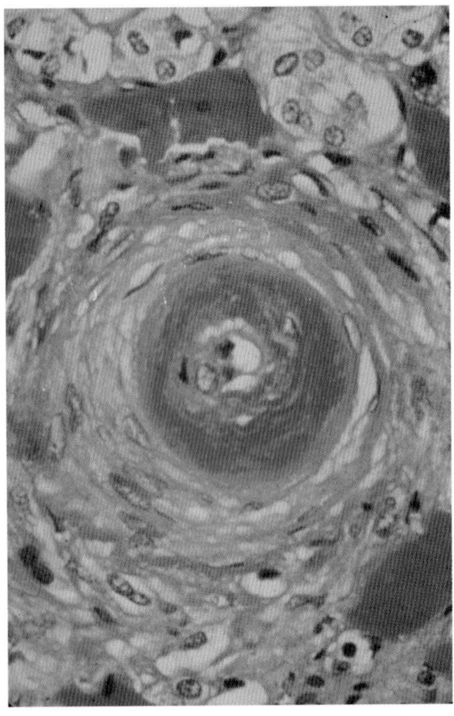

Colour plate 15 Fibrinoid necrosis from accelerated hypertension on a kidney biopsy
(📖 see also p.66)

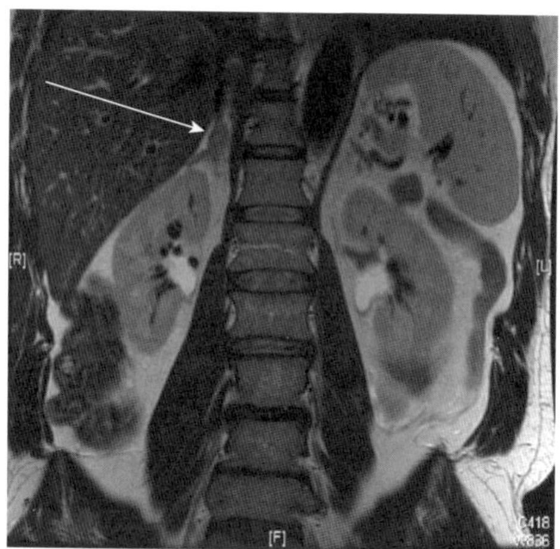

Fig. 4.6 MRI demonstrating a right adrenal adenoma (arrow).

Conn's syndrome

Definition

Conn's syndrome refers to 1° hyperaldosteronism due to an adrenal adenoma. Jerome Conn accurately described the clinical features of such adenomas in 1954, noting the typical hypokalaemia and metabolic alkalosis. The tumour is typically small, <2cm in diameter, and has a 'canary' yellow cut surface (📖 Fig. 4.7).

Secretion of aldosterone by the adenoma is independent of plasma volume or sodium, and in most patients (80%) is unresponsive to angiotensin II. It is strongly dependent on ACTH, but displays incomplete suppression with dexamethasone, in contrast to glucocorticoid remediable hyperaldosteronism.

Demographics

Adrenal adenomas are responsible for ~65% of cases of 1° hyperaldosteronism. Figures on the incidence vary greatly, but estimates are 1–5% of hypertensives. Adenomas are more common in women (2:1) and tend to present in middle-age.

Clinical features

Conn's syndrome usually presents as hypokalaemia in the context of hypertension, or as more severe hypokalaemia after commencing a diuretic. The hypokalaemia may result in symptoms of weakness, lethargy, and paraesthesia. Alternatively, subjects may present with resistant hypertension.

Investigations

- U&Es: ↓ K^+, mild ↑ Na^+, alkalosis. There is often mild hypomagnasaemia and marked urinary K^+ wasting.
- Plasma renin, aldosterone: suppressed renin, ↑ aldosterone, ↑ ARR (📖 see 1° hyperaldosteronism, pp.144–145).
- Failure of salt loading or fludrocortisone to suppress plasma aldosterone (📖 see p.122).
- Adrenal vein sampling: lateralization of >2:1 (📖 see Interventional radiology, p.132).
- Imaging CT (📖 Fig. 4.8) or MRI (may not reveal small adenomas).

Treatment

Medical

Medical therapy may be used short term, as a prelude to surgery, to control the BP and correct electrolyte abnormalities, or long term in patients who are unsuitable or unwilling for surgery. Spironolactone is the drug of choice at doses between 25–200mg/day. This is usually sufficient to normalize the serum potassium. The main side effect is breast tenderness, which, if problematic, may necessitate changing to eplerenone. If additional therapy is required a dihydropyridine CCA may be used.

Surgical

The definitive treatment for lateralizable Conn's syndrome is surgical removal of the adrenal gland. This is often undertaken laparoscopically to minimize recovery time, but a formal laparotomy is occasionally required. Although removal invariably cures the biochemical abnormalities, its effect on BP is variable. At 1 year ~60% of subjects are normotensive, falling to ~50% at 5 years. Young patients with a short duration of hypertension and those with a good response to spironolactone are more likely to achieve normotension. Conversely, older subjects with long antecedent histories of hypertension, and those with resistant hypertension, are more likely to require life-long anti-hypertensive therapy. U&Es should be closely monitored in the postoperative period, although hypomineralocorticodism is rare.

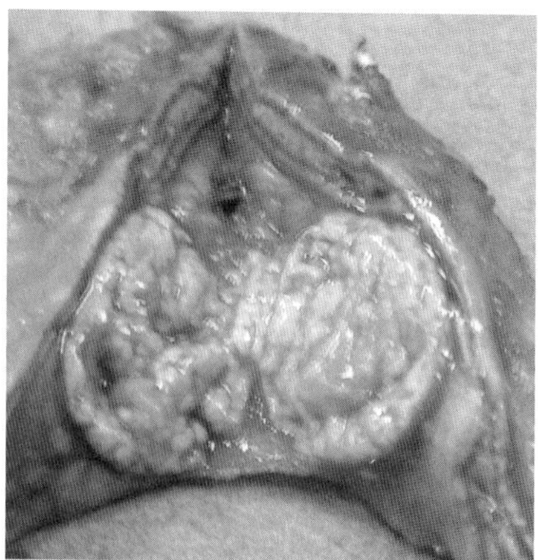

Fig. 4.7 Example of a Conn's tumour (see also Colour plate 10).

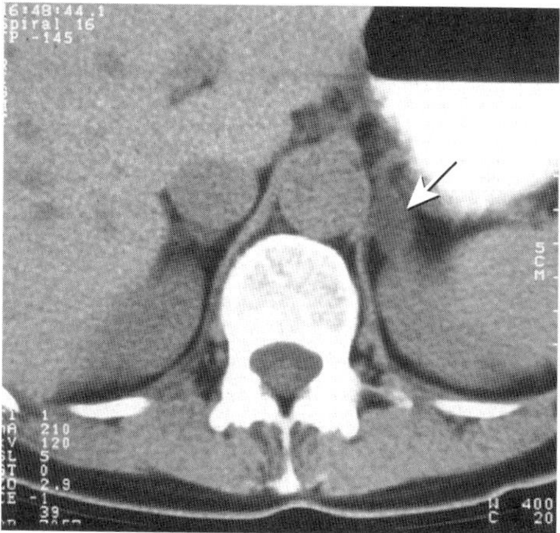

Fig. 4.8 Example of a left adrenal adenoma (arrow). Note: the classical olive shape and low attenuation.

Bilateral adrenal hyperplasia

Definition

Bilateral adrenal hyperplasia (BAH) refers to the syndrome of 1° hyperaldosteronism in the presence of bilateral adrenal gland hyperplasia, which may be micro- or macronodular. However, there is no discrete or lateralizing adenoma identifiable. BAH is synonymous with idiopathic aldosteronism.

Demographics

The quoted proportion of 1° hyperaldosteronism due to BAH, varies greatly from 10–80%. However, with better imaging techniques it is estimated it account for ~25%. BAH is more common in men (4:1), and has a peak incidence of ~60 years.

Investigations

The biochemical abnormalities are usually milder than in Conn's syndrome, with less hypokalaemia and renin suppression. The ARR is invariably elevated, and screening tests positive, but there is a failure of lateralization on venous sampling, and imaging is either normal or displays bulky glands bilaterally (Fig. 4.9). The degree of nodularity varies considerably.

Treatment

Surgery is inappropriate, and the mainstay of therapy is spironolactone. However, it is often insufficient to control the BP alone, and addition of other agents, particularly CCAs, is required. Eplerenone or amiloride may be useful in subjects unable to tolerate doses of spironolactone, which is more common if higher doses are required.

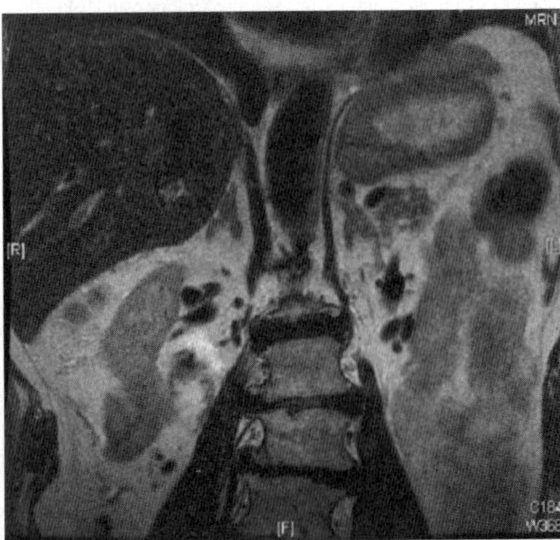

Fig. 4.9 BAH in a 67-year-old man with resistant hypertension.

Cushing's syndrome

Hypertension and hypokalaemia are common presenting features of Cushing's syndrome, particularly when due to ectopic ACTH production. Plasma renin activity and aldosterone levels are usually normal in Cushing's disease, and are often suppressed with ectopic ACTH production. The mechanism of hypertension is complex, and relates to a number of different effects of cortisol. There is up-regulation of angiotensin II signalling and also α-adrenoceptors in vascular tissue. Chronic exposure to excess cortisol leads to a depolarization of smooth muscle cells and an ↑ in intra-cellular calcium content, all favouring vasoconstriction. The very high levels of cortisol found with ectopic ACTH production may also exceed the capacity of the protective 11-β-hydroxysteroid dehydrogenase type II enzyme and result in apparent mineralocorticoid excess and volume retention.

Investigations

- U&Es frequently reveal hypokalaemia, metabolic acidosis, and ↑ glucose.
- Screening for suspected Cushing's syndrome can be undertaken with 24-h urinary cortisol estimation or an overnight dexamethasome suppression test.
- A number of confirmatory tests are available, including low dose dexamethasone suppression, cortisol profiling, and estimation of plasma ACTH.
- Imaging can then be used to provide localization.

Treatment

The standard therapy is surgical excision of the source of ACTH or adrenal tumour. Radiotherapy and medical treatment are useful in non-operable cases or with metastatic spread.

Phaeochromocytoma

Definition

Phaeochromocytomas are rare chromaffin cell tumours that secrete catecholamine, which may produce life-threatening hypertension, dysrhythmias, and heart failure. The majority (90%) are located in the adrenal gland. Extra-adrenal phaeochromocytomas (also called paragangliomas) may be located in a variety of places including the organ of Zuckerkandl, bladder wall, heart, mediastinum, and carotid and jugular bodies, but the majority are intra-abdominal. Overall ~10% are bilateral or multiple.

Adrenal tumours (especially smaller ones) may secrete both NE and epinephrine as they are exposed to high local levels of cortisol necessary to induce transcription of the enzyme phenylethanolamine N-methyltransferase (📖 Fig. 1.6). Nevertheless, noradrenaline secretion usually predominates, except in the case of some familial tumours. Extra-adrenal tumours only secrete NE. Phaeochromocytomas may occasionally also secrete peptides including calcitonin gene-related peptide (CGRP), vasoactive intestinal peptide (VIP), and neuropeptide Y (NPY).

The vast majority of phaeochromocytomas are benign (📖 Fig. 4.10), but up to 10% are malignant. This is more likely with extra-adrenal tumours and those associated with familial syndromes. Defining malignancy is difficult as there is no clear-cut histopathological or biochemical features. In many cases only the presence of metastases allows differentiation.

Demographics

Prevalence estimates are ~0.1–0.5% of hypertensive patients, with an equal gender distribution. The peak age of onset is 30–50 years, but ~10% occur in children, in whom they are more likely to be extra-adrenal or bilateral. The majority of tumours are sporadic, but ~10% are familial (autosomal dominant) or associated with familial syndromes including multiple endocrine neoplasia, and neurofibromatosis (📖 Table 4.2 and Colour plate 13).

Clinical features

Phaechromocytomas may be asymptomatic (50% are discovered incidentally at autopsy), and not all are associated with hypertension. Symptoms are common, but are often nebulous or intermittent, and mimic a variety of other diseases:

- Hypertension: 80% (~1/4 paroxysmal).
- Headache: 80%.
- Palpitations: 70%.
- Sweating: 50%.
- Nausea: 30%.
- Flushing, panic attacks, postural hypotension, diabetes.

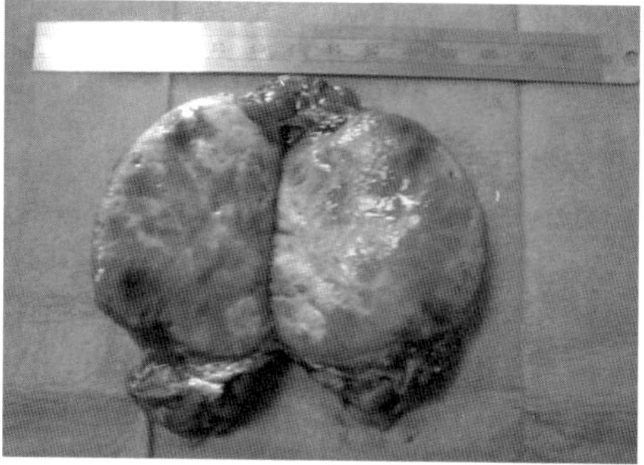

Fig. 4.10 Example of a benign phaeochromocytoma (see also Colour plate 12).

Table 4.2 Familial association of phaeochromocytoma

Syndrome	Risk %	Location	Gene
MEN-2A	50	Adrenal	RET proto-oncogene
MEN-2B	50	Adrenal	RET proto-oncogene
Neurofibromatosis -1	1	Adrenal/abdominal	NF1
Von Hippel–Lindau-2	10–20	Adrenal/abdominal	VHL tumour suppressor
Familial paraganglioma	20	Head and neck/ adrenal	Succinate dehydrogenase

Data from Dluhy RG (2002). Pheochromocytoma—Death of an axiom. *NEJM* **346**:1486.

Investigations

Screening tests should be performed in all those suspected of having a phaeochromocytoma, and is also routinely undertaken in all *de novo* hypertensive in some centres. If these are positive, confirmatory tests may then be performed, and finally the tumour localized by imaging or venous sampling. Genetic testing should be offered for those with a positive family history, children, and those with recurrent tumours.

Screening

Traditionally, urinary VMA was used for screening; this has a very high specificity (96%), but low sensitivity (70%). However, more sensitive tests (~98%) are now available, including urinary fractionated metanephrines and plasma metanephrines. Although this means fewer phaeochromocytomas are missed, this is at the expense of more false positives. In tumours that secrete intermittently it may be necessary to repeat the screening test during symptoms.

In subjects with very high catecholamine metabolite levels, the diagnosis is rarely in doubt and one may move directly to localization. However, confirmatory test are usually indicated if levels are only marginally raised. This usually takes the form of the pentolinium or clonidine suppression test (see Clonidine suppression test, p.120). Failure of suppression of plasma catecholamines (or normetanephrine) is indicative of a phaeochromocytoma.

Localization

This should only be performed once a biochemical diagnosis is made. CT or MRI may be used (Fig. 4.11); the latter has the advantage that contrast agents are less likely to provoke a hypertensive crisis and thus prophylactic α-blockade is not generally required. This is often coupled with isotope scans to delineate uptake into any mass lesion, but may not be needed if there is a high clinical suspicion, unequivocal biochemistry, and a well-defined mass. Traditionally, ^{123}I-MIBG has been used, but not all tumours take this up, and alternatives include ^{111}In-octreotide scanning, or PET with ^{18}F-DOPA or ^{18}F-FDG. PET has better sensitivity and provides better confirmation of likely metastases. Although rarely performed now, plasma catecholamine sampling along the venous tree may be helpful in identified small extra-adrenal tumours in usual locations.

Treatment

It is vital to ensure adequate α-blockade prior to surgery, usually with the irreversible, long-acting antagonist phenoxybenzamine. The usual starting dose is 10mg bd, and the dose is ↑ until there is adequate control of BP and symptoms. This should be initiated a minimum of 7 days before surgery to allow restoration of plasma volume (otherwise severe hypotension can ensure immediately postoperatively). Immediately preoperatively the dose is usually ↑ to produce minimal orthostatic hypotension (fall in SBP of ~20mmHg) to ensure adequate blockade. β-blockade is generally reserved for patients with a resting tachycardia or cardiac disease, and those with significant adrenaline production. This should only be undertaken after adequate α-blockade because of the theoretical risk of blocking β_2-receptor mediated vasodilatation. ^{131}I-MIBG may be used to irradiate malignant phaeochromocytomas if the tumour takes up the ligand.

Definitive treatment is surgical removal, which may be undertaken via a laparoscopic or open approach. Catecholamines should be assessed ~2 weeks postoperatively, and annually from then on. A minority of individuals will remain hypertensive after removal of the tumour, but they usually are symptom-free and have better BP control.

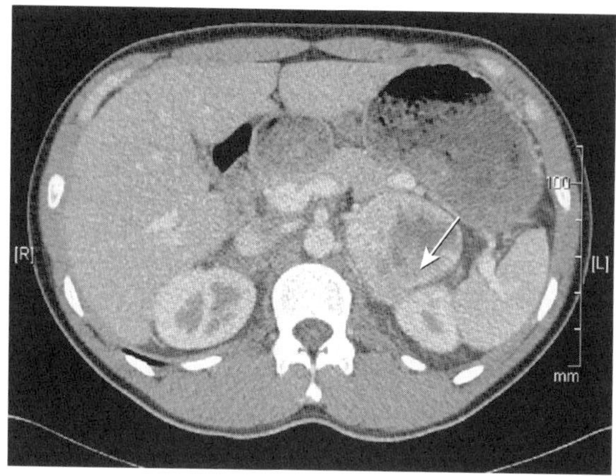

Fig. 4.11 CT of a large mixed density left adrenal phaeochromocytoma (arrow).

Hyperparathyroidism

Hypertension occurs in 30–50% of patients with hyperparathyrodism. The exact mechanism is unclear and may reflect an interplay of factors, including direct vascular effects of calcium and PTH and activation of the renin–angiotensin system, with elevated circulating aldosterone levels. Treatment should be directed at surgical cure of the condition, although only ~20% of patients are rendered normotensive despite a biochemical 'cure'.

Hyperthyroidism

Hypertension has a prevalence of ~25% in patients with hyperthyroidism, and is relatively more prevalent in younger subjects. The usual pattern is systolic hypertension and a widened pulse pressure due to an ↑ cardiac output and plasma volume. PVR tends to be ↓ giving rise to a hyperdynamic circulation. Plasma renin activity tends to be ↑ and there is ↑ sensitivity to catecholamines.

Initial treatment with β-blockade is useful in controlling BP and symptoms, while definitive treatment to produce euthyroidism is introduced. The majority of patients become normotensive after correction of the hyperthyroidism.

Renal parenchymal disease

The association between renal disease and hypertension is strong—renal disease is implicated as the cause or effect of poorly controlled hypertension in up to 5% of cases. The Multiple Risk Factor Intervention Trial (MRFIT)[1] showed that BP is a strong, independent risk factor for the risk of progression to ESRD. Salt and water homeostasis is presumed to be the main determinant of this, although other mechanisms in the pathophysiology are implicated as discussed in the rest of this section. Glomerular disease (glomerulonephritis) and renal ischaemia (renovascular hypertension—📖 see Renal artery stenosis, p.138) are the 2 main underlying pathologies in renal parenchymal disease. Other causes include chronic pyelonephritis and analgesic nephropathy.

Salt sensitivity and RAAS

The pressure response to salt loading or depletion determines the salt sensitivity of that individual—although this is uniformly distributed as a continuous variable in humans. The 1° determinant of this response seems to lie within renal regulation of salt; this is seen when salt-sensitive (SS) rodents become salt resistant (SR) when transplanted with SR kidneys and vice versa.

The interplay between regulatory systems makes interpretation of the cause more difficult; for example, the RAAS can be stimulated or inhibited depending on the state of salt depletion or loading respectively. Aldosterone *per se* has been implicated in the development of glomerular damage independent of the renin–angiotensin system—such that co-administration of an ACEI in animal models does not prevent nephrosclerosis.

Sympathetic nervous system

Plasma noradrenaline is dependent on GFR, so the causal relationship between the role of the sympathetic system in the pathogenesis of hypertension in renal failure is difficult to disentangle; however, other methods of assessing sympathetic activity point to an activation of this system in renal failure. This may partly explain why sympathetic blockade is more effective in end-stage dialysis patients compared to normal subjects. The underlying cause of this may the activation of renal chemo- and baroreceptors resulting in ↑ noradrenergic activity via efferent sympathetic pathways.

Endothelial dysfunction

NO production results in vasodilatation. The role of NO inhibition through substances such as asymmetric dimethylarginine and N-monomethyl-L-arginine (which accumulate in uraemia) has been postulated as another mechanism through which renal impairment results in hypertension. Additionally, production of reactive oxygen species has been implicated in uraemic hypertension which was then reversed by antioxidant therapy.

Erythropoietin

Some renal patients treated with erythropoietin develop hypertension, which may be due to an exaggerated rise in total peripheral resistance or a lack or reduction in cardiac output in response to the correction of anaemia via volume and haematocrit. This may suggest a renal origin to the induction/exacerbation of hypertension in such individuals.

Renal tumours

Whilst hypernephromas (renal cell adenocarcinomas) are reasonably common (especially in an older patient) and rarely linked to ↑BP, the specific renin-secreting tumours *per se*, such as reninomas, are relatively uncommon but closely associated with ↑BP. These are very rare tumours associated with hypokalaemia and high renin. This may be difficult to distinguish in the presence of drugs which raise renin (although a lack of suppression of renin on β-blockade alone in a compliant patient could raise the suspicion), or in other cases of 2° hypertension due to renal ischaemia, e.g. RAS.

Most renin-secreting tumours present as severe hypertension in a relatively younger population <30 years of age (prevalence approximately 0.03% amongst hypertensive patients).

Renal cell carcinomas present as an incidental finding during routine scanning or with symptoms, although usually this occurs only when the disease is advanced. It affects a predominantly older patient cohort. Lymphatic and haematogenous routes result in metastases to bones, liver, and lungs.

Clinical features

- Hypertension in young age—for reninoma.
- Hypokalaemia.
- Tumour haemorrhage—flank pain, anaemia, and hypotension.

Investigations

- U&Es.
- Renin—this is sometimes normal with a very high pro-renin level
- USS renal
- CT abdomen.
- Selective renin vein sampling—for reninoma.
- IV urography—now rarely performed.

Treatment is by surgical removal of the tumour.

Diabetic nephropathy

As the incidence of diabetes and the obesity epidemic rises, concomitantly there has been a rise in the incidence of diabetic nephropathy. Optimal glucose and BP control in this high risk group is vital to reduce TOD—which ultimately results in glomerulosclerosis. The mechanism is that of reduced renal blood flow presumed to be due to ↑ glomerular afferent resistance—resulting in ↑ efferent vasoconstriction and glomerular hyperfiltration. This progresses to glomerulosclerosis, leading to microalbuminuria, and finally frank proteinuria (📖 see also Diabetes, p.196).

Treatment

Salt restriction is advised but not always adhered to, necessitating the use of loop diuretics in most renal failure patients. Ultimately, tight control of BP ameliorates against declining renal function—the current targets for BP control in renal patients are lower (akin to those with CVD or diabetes) at <130/80mmHg.

Thiazide diuretics are ineffective in patients in poor renal function—unlike loop diuretics which can ameliorate fluid overload and BP. Large single doses of loop diuretics may be required (up to 250mg of furosemide), titrating to effect in terms of urine output, and if this is ineffective in producing a natriuresis, the dose frequency can be ↑, monitoring for toxicity throughout. CCAs, α-blockers, and minoxidil have been found to be useful in renal patients also.

The renoprotective effects of ACEI to prevent progression to frank proteinuria especially in diabetic populations is discussed in 📖 Diabetes, p.196.

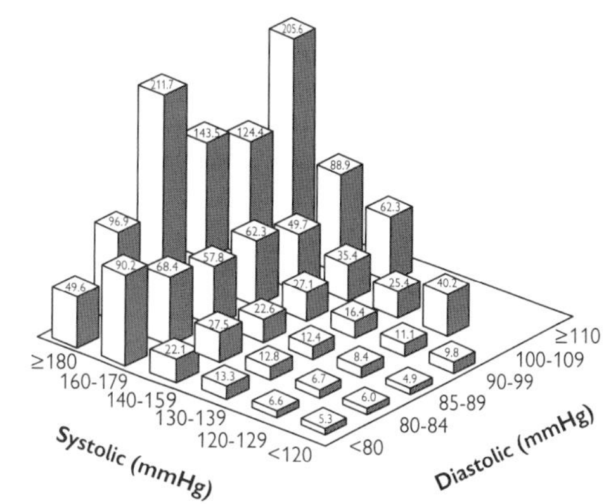

Fig. 4.12 MRFIT graph showing progression to ESRD increases with increasing BP. Reproduced with permission from Klag MJ *et al.* (1996). Blood pressure and end-stage renal disease in men. *NEJM* **334:** 13–8.

Reference

1. Klag MJ, *et al.* (1996). Blood pressure and end-stage renal disease in men. *NEJM* **334**:13–8.

Adult polycystic kidney disease

Definition

Adult polycystic kidney disease (APKD) is an autosomal dominant disorder in which there is progressive focal cyst formation and dilatation in the kidneys and other organs. It is the commonest genetic cause of renal failure. Conversely, the autosomal recessive polycystic kidney disease is the commonest inheritable cause of renal cysts in early childhood.

Up to 1/3 of patients <50 years newly diagnosed with APKD are found to be hypertensive; this ↑ depending on the age at presentation or diagnosis. This can occur despite having normal renal function but is commoner in those with a mutation at the *PKD1* locus on chromosome 16.

There is a school of thought suggesting that ↑ renin production contributes to the pathogenesis of hypertension in APKD.

Demographics

APKD is more severe in males compared to females. It accounts for up to 10% of cases of ESRD in the Western hemisphere. 90% of the cases are due to a mutation in *PKD1* and the rest to *PKD2* or *PKD3*.

Clinical features

- Abdominal pain.
- Haematuria.
- Hypertension.
- Renal failure.
- Strokes—a small proportion associated with intracranial aneurysms.

Investigations

- U&Es.
- Urine microalbuminuria.
- Urine dipstick for blood and protein.
- Renin and aldosterone levels.
- 24-h urine for proteinuria.
- Renal ultrasound.
- Creatinine clearance, e.g. ethylenediamine tetra-acetic acid (EDTA) clearance.
- Genetic testing and counselling.

The clinical diagnosis is usually established on history and ultrasound examination. A genetic locus may be pursued in the index case in order to determine if screening of family members is required.

Treatment

CCAs, ARAs, and ACEIs have a more pronounced effect in patients with APKD. The role of renin inhibition in these patients is yet to be determined. Ultimately good BP control minimizes the risk of CV complications as in any other group. Genetic screening after proper counselling helps identify and follow-up cohorts in a more coherent manner to reduce the risk of events.

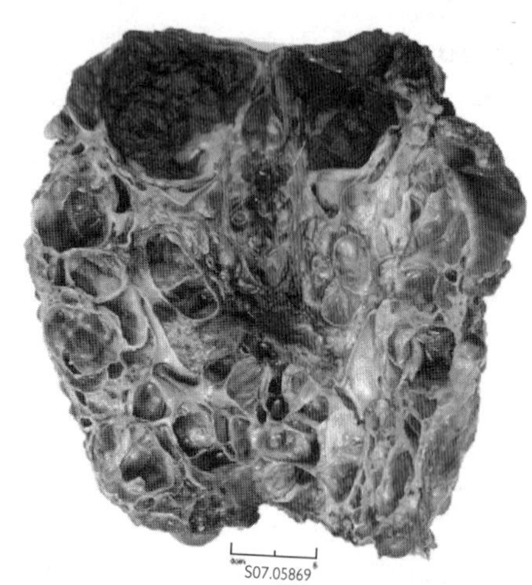

Fig. 4.13 A macroscopic view of a polycystic kidney (📖 see also Colour plate 14).

Liquorice

Liquorice is commonly found in liquorice sweets and is extensively used in food and tobacco products as well as herbal remedies. It has mineralocorticoid and glucocorticoid properties. The glycyrrhetinic acid component of liquorice causes hypertension and hypokalaemia through a mineralocorticoid effect by inhibiting 11-β-hydroxysteroid dehydrogenase (type 2), which inactivates cortisol. This is more so in chronic liquorice ingestion as opposed to any acute intake. The biochemical picture is one of low serum potassium associated with low renin and aldosterone levels, ↑ urinary free cortisol, ↑ cortisol:cortisone ratio, and raised urinary potassium. Rhabdomyolysis and myoglobinuria may occur through hypokalaemia as a result of poisoning. Potassium supplementation and hydration ± urine alkalinization may be required. The hypertension reverses on withdrawal of liquorice.

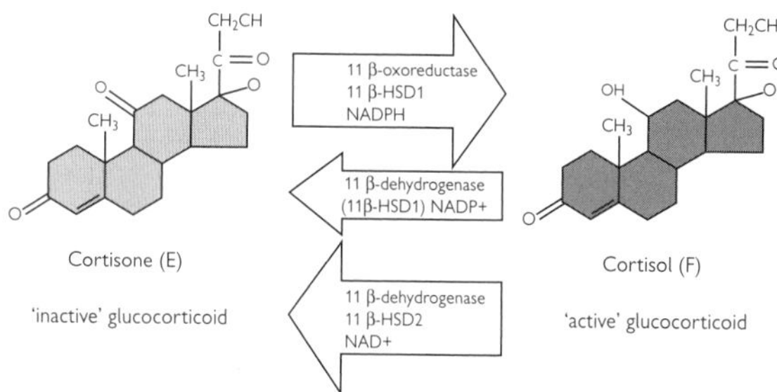

Fig. 4.14 11 β-hydroxysteroid dehydrogenase and its effects on glucocorticoids. 11β-HSD, 11 β-hydroxysteroid dehydrogenase; NADP, nicotinamide adenine diphosphate; NADPH, nicotinamide adenine diphosphate (reduced).

Alcohol

Observational data point to the link between chronic excess alcohol consumption and the development of hypertension and other CV disorders. Low to moderate intake, however, is associated with a better CV outcome. Binge drinking is associated with a worse outcome, but generally patients should be advised to adhere to recommended alcohol targets and to drink in moderation. Whilst the underlying mechanisms are unclear, this may be through activation of the sympathetic nervous system, ↑ cortisol secretion, or altered insulin sensitivity.

Whilst causal links are not fully established, a reduction in intake has demonstrated, at best, a 5 to 8/3mmHg reduction in pressures—this is evidenced from meta-analyses of RCTs (📖 Fig. 4.15).

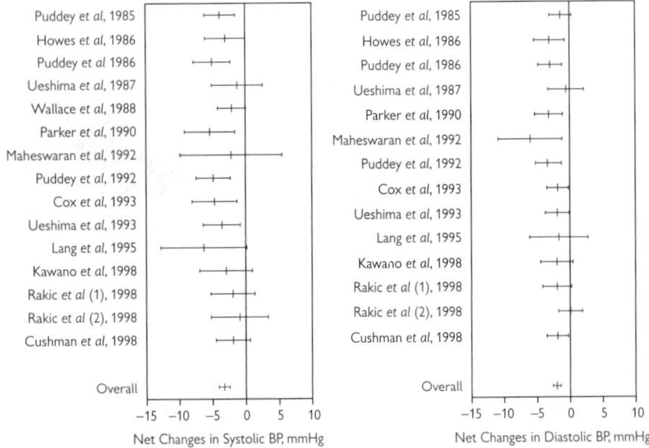

Fig. 4.15 Net change in BP after alcohol reduction across 15 RCTs (with corresponding 95% confidence intervals). Reproduced with permission from Xin X, *et al.* (2001). Effects of alcohol reduction on blood pressure: a meta-analysis of randomized controlled trials. *Hypertension* **38**:1112–17.

ocaine

ocaine use is associated with hypertension via its action of facilitatir techolamine release and inhibiting uptake 1 at the sympathetic nerv ereby resulting in adrenergic hypersensitivity. It also blocks voltag ted sodium channels thereby working as a local anaesthetic. Patien ay present with tachycardia (β-receptor stimulation) and hypertensic x-adrenergic receptor via noradrenaline) and associated complicatio ncluding ischaemic chest pain (coronary vasospasm), acute coronary sy romes, dysrhythmias, cardiac arrest, aortic dissection, dyspnoea, pne nomediastinum, seizures, headaches, anxiety, extrapyramidal reactior habdomyolysis, bowel infarction, and so on. Chronic use is associate with premature atherosclerosis.

Management in the acute setting includes methods of active elimination (l preventing absorption), using benzodiazepines for seizures (and excludi intracerebral events) – this may relieve some of the hypertension and a tation. Alternatively, vasodilators such as nitrates, sodium nitroprussi or α-blockers may be used. β-blockers are best avoided as they wors coronary spasm and promote unmitigated α-adrenergic actions such worsening hypertension.

Heavy metals

Heavy metals such as lead, cadmium, and arsenic can result in hyperte sion through a variety of mechanisms. Cadmium is possibly thought cause a disruption to normal angiogenesis. Arsenic causes an ↑ in o dative stress through the production of reactive oxidative species. Le exposure is thought to worsen endothelial function by impairing NO pr duction and stimulating the RAAS system. The evidence linking these hypertension is, at best, modest.

Oral contraceptive pill

Shortly after its widespread introduction in the 1960s, it became apparent that the combined OCP was associated with the development of hypertension in some women. Despite the considerable reduction in oestrogen content of modern pills this link remains. In contrast, there does not seem to be any association between the progesterone-only-pill ('mini pill') and hypertension.

Overall, there is a modest ~2/1mmHg ↑ in BP in women taking the combined OCP. Physiologically, this is due to an expansion of plasma volume and ↑ cardiac output. However, a significant minority of women have a much larger ↑ in BP. This usually occurs in the 1st few months, and is reversible if the drug is withdrawn. However, the risk of developing hypertension in the longer term is also ~2-fold elevated, and is significantly higher in older or obese women and those with borderline hypertension. The combined OCP should not be prescribed to women who are already hypertensive and regular BP checks are advised for women who are taking it.

Steroids

The link between steroids and hypertension is probably best explained from its mineralocorticoid action to promote salt and water retention, which is more marked at higher doses. However, there is some suggestion that glucocorticoids have direct actions on both glucocorticoid and mineralocorticoid receptors in CV tissues via the 11 β-hydroxysteroid dehydrogenase enzyme. This is similar to the effects seen in Cushing's syndrome (📖 see Cushing's syndrome, p.151) and in the syndrome of apparent mineralocorticoid excess (AME). Long-term, high-dose steroid therapy is associated with a number of adverse events—and should therefore be discouraged. In patients who do not have the option, CV risk (in particular BP) should be monitored closely and intervention taken sooner rather than later. Diuretics may be useful for salt and water retention.

Non-steroidal anti-inflammatory drugs

The association between NSAIDs and hypertension has come from changes noted from a variety of studies. Some NSAIDs are more culpable than others—in particular, naproxen and indometacin. The mechanism is thought to be due to cyclo-oxygenase (COX) inhibition and a reduction in prostaglandin synthesis, which are vasodilatory. There is also some evidence to suggest COX-2 inhibitors cause poorer BP control when compared with COX-1 inhibitors. Salt and water retention and the up-regulation of RAS may also have a part to play in the genesis of hypertension with NSAIDs, especially in at-risk individuals. NSAIDs essentially affect the efficacy of most anti-hypertensive agents; therefore, their use should be minimized in hypertensive patients.

Immunosuppressives

Cyclosporin-induced hypertension has been well described and is clinically well apparent. This is also true for other calcineurin inhibitors, such as tacrolimus, but to a lesser extent. Whilst sex and race do not seem to play a role, drug dose, age, and pre-existing hypertension predisposes to the development of drug-induced hypertension.

It is thought to be mediated through a myriad of mechanisms including a reduction in nitric oxide production, ↑ thromboxane A2 production, ↓ prostaglandin synthesis and ↑ endothelin release. These result in a volume-dependant hypertension with vasoconstriction at the afferent arteriole. Consequently, drugs which affect low renin hypertension—such as CCAs and diuretic—are most likely to have an impact on BP control.

Vascular endothelial growth factor inhibitors

Vascular endothelial growth factor (VEGF) inhibitors are a new class of agents which act by inhibiting angiogenesis. They are known to cause hypertension in a dose-dependant manner which may resolve on withdrawal of therapy. The mechanisms by which this is thought to occur are not fully established but may include endothelial dysfunction via oxidative stress and a reduction in NO thereby ↑ vascular tone. Other possible mechanisms include microvascular rarefaction, where there is a reduced density of capillaries (also seen in essential hypertension). Whilst the management includes standard antihypertensive therapies (including ACEIs, ARAs, dihydropyridine CCAs, and diuretics), it is unclear if some of these drugs may be more suitable than others due to varying effects on VEGF secretion. Non-dihydropyridine CCAs have a cytochorme p450 interaction with some VEGF inhibitors.

Monoamine oxidase inhibitors

Monoamine oxidase inhibitors (MAOIs) *per se* do not cau
sion—however, if taken together with tyramine-rich foods
Marmite™, wine, chocolate etc.) can result in a 'cheese rea
mode of action as effective antidepressants includes delayin
ytryptophan and sympathomimetic amine metabolism, but als
echolamine stores in the postganglionic neuron. The non-selec
bind irreversibly to MAO A and B, *per se*. However, when co-ing
tyramine-containing foodstuffs or with serotonin inhibitors, they
a tyramine reaction (cheese reaction) which is essentially a hyp
crisis. The tyramine is more bioavailable (due to inhibition of M
the gut mucosa) and causes release of NE from vesicle stores st
post-synaptic α-adrenoceptors and causing vasoconstriction.

This reaction is less likely with the more modern MAOIs which are
ible and specific (e.g. selegiline which is a MAO B inhibitor vs. moclo
which is a short-acting MAO A inhibitor).

More serious than this is the potentially life-threatening serotoni
drome which can occur when MAOIs are combined with other sero
agonists (e.g. tricyclic antidepressants; opioids like pethidine and tram
CNS stimulants, e.g. sibutramine, amphetamines, Ecstasy tablets,
MDMA; triptans used in migraines, etc.). Diagnosis is clinical and seve
is based on the symptoms. It is not the same as neuroleptic malign
syndrome. Treatment includes discontinuation of precipitant therapi
supportive measures, control of seizures, use of serotonin antagonis
and occasionally controlled cooling with paralysis and intubation on a
intensive care unit.

Table 4.3 Classification of the serotonin syndrome

Severity	Symptoms
Mild	Tachycardia
	Shivering
	Sweating
	Myoclonus
	Mydriasis
	Hyper-reflexia
Moderate	Hypertension
	Hyperthermia (>40°C)
	Borborygmi
Severe	Rhabdomyolysis
	Seizures
	Renal failure
	Metabolic acidosis

Chapter 5

Monogenic syndromes

Acknowledgement

We are indebted to Dr Kevin O'Shaughnessy for his help with this chapter.

Introduction

Essential hypertension is most likely the result of a complex gene–environment interaction. The results of genome wide searches to date for the 'underlying' genes in hypertension have been far from fruitful, with the conclusion that essential hypertension probably results from small effects of multiple genetic polymorphisms.

The failure to identify any underlying causes undoubtedly reflects a lack of power of early studies, but also probably a lack of adequately phenotyping subjects. Although we consider essential hypertension as a single disorder, this is clearly far from the truth, and subjects can be subdivided according to a number of pathways, including biochemical, physiological, and pharmacological differences. It is likely that greater emphasis on large, well-phenotyped cohorts may yield novel genetic candidates underlying some of the variability of BP in the population.

In contrast, in a small number of hypertensives, a mutation in a single gene is responsible for their condition. These so-called monogenic syndromes have, as yet, not translated into identifying a cause for essential hypertension. They have highlighted the importance of salt and water handling in the kidney in the genesis of hypertension, and that different pathways may lead to the same disease in outward phenotypic appearance.

However, dissecting the underlying causes of monogenic syndromes in hypertension highlights potential pathways that may yield new therapeutic targets.

Other similar disorders are associated with hypotension or normotension. Nevertheless, these are discussed in this chapter as they help explain the physiology.

Pathophysiology

Salt excess states

Salt excess is characterized by a ↓ renin and ↓ aldosterone profile in combination with ↓ K^+. There are a number of genetic causes of this, including:

- AME.
- Mineralocorticoid receptor-activating mutation.
- Gordon's syndrome.
- Hypertensive congenital adrenal hyperplasia (CAH).
- Glucocorticoid remediable aldosteronism.
- Liddle's syndrome.

All are associated with hypertension. The renin–aldosterone status may provide a clue as to the underlying cause and how to proceed further with the diagnostic test (📖 Fig. 5.1).

Other monogenic syndromes

Some of these syndromes reveal how loop, thiazide, and K^+-sparing diuretics vary in their actions as they affect different parts of the nephron (📖 see Table 5.1 and Fig. 5.2).

For example, loop diuretics block NKCC2 in the ascending limb of the loop of Henle resulting in ↓ K^+, metabolic alkalosis, and fluid loss—similar to the defect seen in Bartter's syndrome.

Thiazides block the NaCl sensitive co-transporter in the apical membrane of the distal convoluted tubule (DCT)—similar to the defect seen in Gitelman's syndrome.

Amiloride blocks the epithelial sodium channel (ENaC) thereby preventing Na^+ reabsorption in the late DCT and cortical collecting duct. In Liddle's syndrome, ENaC activity is ↑ and therefore amiloride is the most effective antihypertensive in this monogenic syndrome.

Table 5.1 Monogenic syndromes affecting the nephron and BP effects

Monogenic syndrome	Anatomical site	BP effect
Bartter's	Thick ascending limb of loop of Henle	↓ BP
Gitelman's	DCT	↓ BP
Liddle's	Collecting duct	↑ BP

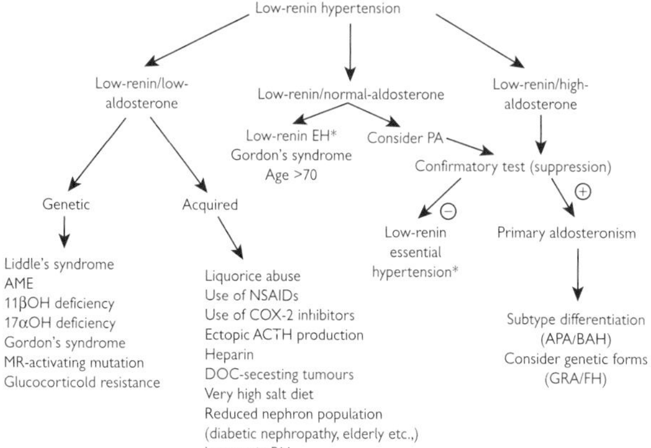

Fig. 5.1 Diagnostic flowchart for low renin hypertension. Adapted with permission from Mulatero P, *et al.* (2007). Diagnosis and treatment of low-renin hypertension. *Clin Endocrinol* **67**:324–34.

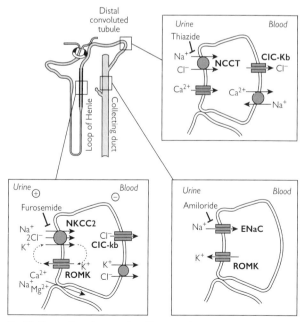

Fig. 5.2 Monogenic syndromes and renal homeostasis.

Apparent mineralocorticoid excess

Prevalence

Very rare: 40 pedigrees worldwide.

Genetic inheritance

Autosomal recessive.

Pathophysiology

The defect causes inactivation of the *11βHSD2* gene which encodes the kidney 11-β-hydroxysteroid dehydrogenase, The enzyme usually deactivates cortisol to the inactive cortisone, thereby protecting the mineralocorticoid receptor from cortisol. A failure to do this results in excess stimulation of the mineralocorticoid receptor by cortisol—leading to ↑ salt and water retention. Liquorice ingestion (also bioflavinoids and carbenoxolone, all of which inhibit 11βHSD2) is an acquired cause of AME (📖 see Liquorice, p.163).

Presentation

It usually presents in early childhood with low renin hypertension.

Biochemistry

- ↓ K^+.
- ↑ Na^+.
- ↓ renin.
- ↓ aldosterone.
- ↑ urinary cortisol/cortisone ratio.

Treatment

- Spironolactone.
- Metyrapone.

Mineralocorticoid receptor-activating mutation

Prevalence

Extremely rare: only 1 family described.

Genetic inheritance

Autosomal dominant.

Pathophysiology

The mutation lies in the mineralocorticoid receptor which causes it to be activated by steroids lacking 21-hydroxyl groups, such as progesterone and spironolactone. Both normally antagonize the receptor but have the opposite effect on this mutant receptor.

Presentation

It usually presents as early onset hypertension in females that is exacerbated in pregnancy due to elevated progesterone levels.

Biochemistry

- ↓ K^+.
- ↓ renin.
- ↓ aldosterone.

Treatment

- Delivery of the fetus.
- Amiloride, in theory, may be useful but spironolactone worsens hypertension.

Gordon's syndrome

Prevalence

Rare.

Genetic inheritance

Autosomal dominant.

Pathophysiology

Also known as pseudohypoaldosteronism type II (PHA2), this is a monogenic syndrome linked to chromosomes 1, 12, and 17 and more recently associated with mutations in 2 kinases called WNK1 and WNK4– wild types usually inhibit the thiazide sensitive NaCL co-transporter (NCCT) but the mutants cause excess Cl^- and Na^+ reabsorption.

Presentation

Hypertension, muscle weakness, and sometimes periodic paralysis. Other features include short stature, mental impairment.

Biochemistry

- ↑ K^+.
- ↓ renin.
- ↓ aldosterone.
- Metabolic acidosis.
- ↑ Cl^-.

Treatment

- Low salt diet.
- Thiazide diuretics.

Hypertensive congenital adrenal hyperplasia

Prevalence

Overall prevalence of CAH is 1 in 16,s000 (higher in some populations: 1 in 400 in Alaska). CYP11B1 accounts for about 5% of all cases of CAH.

Genetic inheritance

Autosomal recessive

Pathophysiology

CAH is a constellation of disorders, only some of which produce hypertension. The 21-hydroxylase deficiency (CYP21A2) is associated with normotension whereas the 11β-hydroxylase (CYP11B1) and 17α-hydroxylase (CYP17) deficiencies leads to excess deoxycorticosterone which causes hypertension through a mineralocorticoid action (📖 see Fig 5.3).

Presentation

- Hypertension.
- Virilization (girls) or precocious puberty (boys)—CYP11B1.
- 1° amenorrhoea, delayed sexual maturation (girls) or ambiguous genitalia (boys)—CYP17.

Biochemistry

- ↓ K^+.
- ↓ renin.
- ↓ aldosterone.

Treatment

- Steroids.

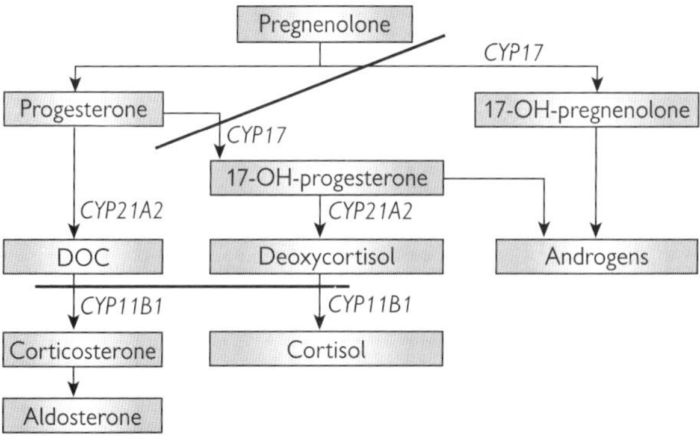

Fig. 5.3 The adrenal steroid pathways. CYP11B1 and CYP17 are associated with hypertension due to excess production of deoxycorticosterone (DOC).

Glucocorticoid remediable aldosteronism

Prevalence

Rare.

Genetic inheritance

Autosomal dominant.

Pathophysiology

Also known as familial hyperaldosteronism type I or glucocorticoid suppressible aldosteronism - wherein ectopic aldosterone synthesis occurs in the zona fasciculata under the direct influence of ACTH rather than the renin–angiotensin feedback system or K^+. It is due to a translocation resulting in a hybrid CYP11B1/CYP11B2 gene. (Familial hyperaldosteronism type II is an autosomal dominant condition not suppressible by dexamethasone.)

Presentation

- Hypertension in youth resistant to standard treatment.
- Haemorrhagic strokes.

Biochemistry

- ↓ K^+.
- ↓ renin.
- ↓ aldosterone.
- Metabolic alkalosis may be present.

Treatment

- Salt restriction.
- Steroids.
- Spironolactone, amiloride, or triamterene.

Liddle's syndrome

Prevalence

Rare.

Genetic inheritance

Autosomal dominant.

Pathophysiology

This is due to a gain-of-function mutation (protein deletion/alteration) at chromosome 16 affecting the β- or γ-subunit of the ENaC channel in the collecting duct of the nephron. This causes ↑ Na^+ reabsorption. The original proband was cured of their hypertension by renal transplantation.

Presentation

- Presents as hypertension in childhood/young adulthood.
- Usually asymptomatic and resistant to standard antihypertensives.

Biochemistry

- ↑ Na^+.
- ↓ K^+.
- Metabolic alkalosis.
- ↓ renin.
- ↓ aldosterone.
- ↓ urine Na^+.

Treatment

- Low salt diet.
- K^+-sparing diuretics, e.g. amiloride, triamterene which block ENaC (not spironolactone).

Bartter's syndrome

Prevalence

1 in 1 million.

Genetic inheritance

Autosomal recessive.

Pathophysiology

There are 4 different types described. The genetic defect in classical Bartter's (type 3) causes a failure in active Cl^- reabsorption in the ascending limb of the loop of Henle. The missense mutation in the gene, however, may be in the one of a few locations which differentiates the different subytypes of Bartter's as listed in 📖 Table 5.2.

Presentation

- Neonatal/infancy: polyhydramnios, prematurity.
- Early childhood: dehydration, nephrocalcinosis, renal stones, failure to thrive, renal failure.
- Polyuria and polydipsia are common.
- Weakness, muscle cramps, abdominal pain.
- Type 4 Bartter's may present with sensorineural deafness as the defect affects a similar channel in the inner ear.
- Low to normal BP.

Biochemistry

- ↓ K^+.
- Metabolic alkalosis.
- ↑ renin.
- ↑ aldosterone.
- ↑ urinary excretion of Na^+, K^+, Mg^{2+}, Cl^-, and Ca^{2+}.

Treatment

- ↑ salt in diet (both Na+ and K+).
- K+ supplementation.
- Spironolactone.
- Non-steroidal anti-inflammatory agents.
- ACEIs.

Table 5.2 Subtypes of Bartter's syndrome

Type	Channel affected	Location	Effect in normal state
1	NKCC2	Apical surface of ascending loop of Henle	Transport Na^+, K^+, $2Cl^-$ from ECF to cell
2	ROMK	Apical surface of ascending loop of Henle	Transport K^+ out of cells
3	CLCNKB	Basolateral surface of loop of Henle	Cl^- transport
4	BSND (co-factor for CLC-KB in ear and kidney)	Basolateral surface of DCT	Cl^- transport

Gitelman's syndrome

Incidence

1 in 40,000, prevalence of heterozygotes is ~1% in Caucasians. One of the commonest inherited tubular disorders.

Genetic inheritance

Autosomal recessive.

Pathophysiology

Mutation affecting SLC12A3 encoding the NCCT (thiazide-sensitive NCCT) in the DCT. It is a milder disease than Bartter's.

Presentation

- Presents in early childhood late childhood or adulthood.
- Muscle weakness, tetany, paresthesiae, joint problems, vomiting, abdominal pain.
- Hypokalaemia periodic paralysis.
- Prolonged QTc.
- May be normo- or hypotensive.

Biochemistry

- ↓ K^+, ↓ Mg^{2+}.
- Metabolic alkalosis.
- ↓ urinary Ca^{2+}, ↑ urinary Mg^{2+}.

Treatment

- ↑ salt in diet (both Na+ and K+).
- Mg2+ and K+ supplementation.
- Amiloride.

Chapter 6

Special populations

Pregnancy

Hypertension in the context of pregnancy is relatively common, affecting ~15% of all pregnancies. Although usually uncomplicated, it may occur in the context of pre-eclampsia. Maternal hypertension is the 2nd most common cause of maternal deaths in the UK. Therefore, close monitoring and co-operation between medical specialties is essential. It is also important to recognize that treatment differs from standard practice.

Measuring BP

BP should be recorded in a seated position using Korotkoff I and V. The routine use of Korotkoff 4 for diastolic pressure has been abandoned because V is more reliably detected and closer to true diastolic pressure. In the very few women in whom sounds can be heard down to zero, Korotkoff IV should be used, but this must be recorded in the notes. Generally, mercury devices are preferred as many oscillometric devices have not been validated in pregnant women. Aneroid devices should be avoided.

Haemodynamic changes in pregnancy

Pregnancy is associated with a number of dramatic changes in the CV system that come about to meet the ↑ metabolic demands of the mother and fetus. Over the course of a normal pregnancy, circulating blood volume ↑ steadily to ~150% of normal by term. PVR falls until mid gestation and then gradually returns to normal by term (📖 Fig. 6.1). Cardiac output ↑ by 50% over the first 20 weeks of gestation, and then plateaus until delivery. This is driven by an ↑ in heart rate throughout pregnancy and a marked ↑ in stroke volume during the 1st trimester. The overall effect is that BP tends to fall from conception until mid-pregnancy and then returns to normal by term. This pattern of haemodynamic changes is different in women who develop hypertension during pregnancy, and varies depending upon the nature of the underlying condition (📖 Fig. 6.1).

Definitions

Hypertension in pregnancy is defined as a BP consistently (2 or more occasions) >140/90mmHg. Some units also based their definition on a single diastolic pressure over 110mmHg, or a rise of 15mmHg in diastolic or 30mmHg systolic from booking. However, the validity of such approaches is unclear. Hypertension in pregnancy can be divided into 3 main categories (📖 Fig. 6.2):

- ***Chronic hypertension*** defined as an elevated BP at conception or prior to 20 weeks' gestation—usually 'essential' in nature.
- ***Gestational or pregnancy-associated hypertension*** also referred to as non-proteinuric pregnancy-induced hypertension (PIH). Defined as an elevated BP after 20 weeks *without* significant proteinuria.
- ***Pre-eclampsia (toxaemia)*** or proteinuric PIH (PPIH). Defined as an elevation in BP after 20 weeks' gestation *with* significant proteinuria (≥1+ on dipsick, or 300mg/24h).

► The term PIH encompasses gestational hypertension and pre-eclampsia, the distinction being whether or not there is significant proteinuria.

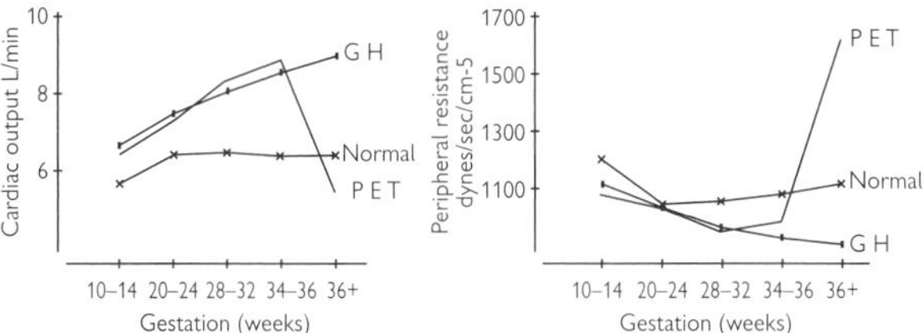

Fig. 6.1 Changes in cardiac output and peripheral resistance in normal pregnancy and women who develop pre-eclampsia (PET) or pregnancy associated (gestational; GH) hypertension. Redrawn with permission from Bosio PM, *et al.* (1999). Maternal central hemodynamics in hypertensive disorders of pregnancy. *Obstet Gynecol* **94**:978–84.

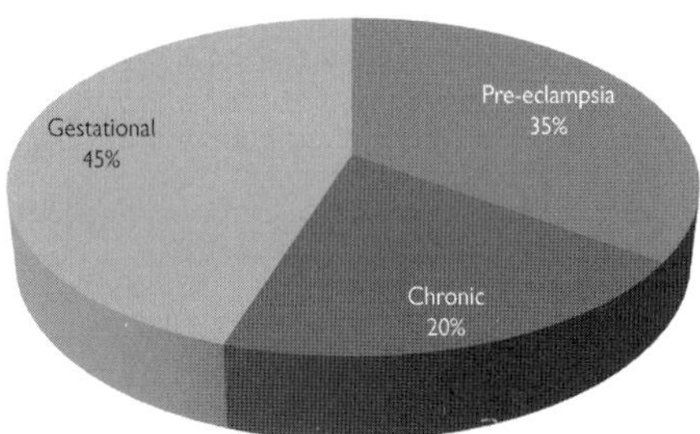

Fig. 6.2 The relative frequencies of the 3 types of hypertension in pregnancy.

Antihypertensive drugs therapy

Given the potential for adverse effect to both the mother and foetus the use of any drug in a pregnant woman is a balance between risk and benefit. Perhaps unsurprisingly, most antihypertensive agents are unlicensed for use in pregnancy because safety and efficacy studies have not been undertaken. Thus older agents, that were widely used before concerns about teratogenicty were raised, tend to be the only agents with 'proven' safety records. The main aim of treating hypertension is to prevent the development of severe hypertension. There appears to be little effect on other outcome measures in mild/moderate hypertension.

Methydopa

Widely used in pregnancy; acts to reduce sympathetic outflow by a central mechanism. Placebo-controlled trials have confirmed the efficacy of methyldopa in reducing BP, but other beneficial effects seem small. Side-effects such as depression and sedation are its major drawbacks. Long-term follow-up studies have shown that methyldopa is not associated with any risk of teratogenicity. The usual dose range is 200mg–1g, 2–3 times daily.

β-blockers

These agents are widely used in pregnancy, and controlled trials confirm their efficacy. Labetalol (also has α-blocking effects) is licensed in pregnancy and has a favourable safety and side-effect profile (care in asthmatics). Atenolol has been associated with a fall in placental perfusion and reduced fetal growth in older studies and should be avoided (the effects of newer agents are unclear). The usual dose of labetaolol is 100–400mg, 2 or 3 times a day (maximum dose 2.4g daily).

CCAs

A range of agents have been used in pregnancy and data suggests that they are at least as effective as other agents in reducing BP. Nifedipine is the most widely used and has a good safety profile, and amlodipine is probably also safe. Nifedipine should not be used in the short-acting form, especially in severe hypertension; usual dose 20–90mg daily.

Other agents

Thiazide diuretics have fallen out of favour in pregnancy, particularly in pre-eclampsia which is often associated with a reducing in plasma volume. However, early studies suggested that thiazides were effective and showed similar safety to other antihypertensives. Nevertheless, they cannot be currently recommended. ACEIs are teratogenic even in the early phases of pregnancy[1] and should therefore be avoided from the outset, as should ARAs. α-blockers may be used in more resistant cases.

Targets

There is no clear evidence about acceptable BP targets in pregnancy. Recently there have been concerns regarding excessive reduction in BP leading to fetal growth restriction (📖 Fig. 6.3). Moreover, although antihypertensive drugs may prevent the development of severe hypertension in women with mild–moderate BP elevation, they do not seem to improve other aspects of maternal or fetal outcomes. Thus excessive BP lowering should be avoided, and reasonable target pressures are 130–150/80–100mmHg.

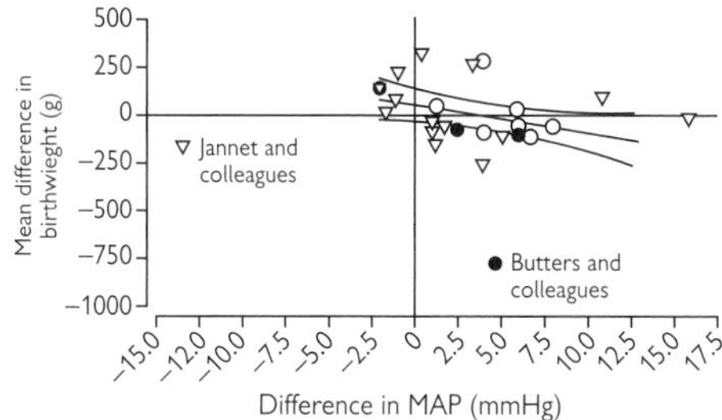

Fig. 6.3 Relationship between fall in MAP and birth weight. Redrawn from von Dadelszen P, *et al.* (2000). Fall in mean arterial pressure and fetal growth restriction in pregnancy hypertension: a meta-analysis. *Lancet* **355**:87–92, © 2000, with permission from Elsevier.

Reference

1. Cooper WO, *et al.* (2006). Major congenital malformations after first-trimester exposure to ACE inhibitors. *NEJM* **354**:2443–51.

Pregnancy: chronic hypertension

Chronic hypertension complicates ~3% of all pregnancies. The vast majority of chronic hypertension in pregnancy is 1° or essential hypertension. 2° hypertension is rare, accounting for <2% of all cases. Occasionally 2° hypertension may be diagnosed *de novo* in pregnancy; the most frequent cause being intrinsic renal disease. It is important to exclude phaeochromocytoma to avoid the potentially devastating consequences during later pregnancy. Chronic hypertension in pregnancy is more likely in older, obese, or black women, and those with pre-existing CV or renal disease.

Risks

Chronic hypertension is associated with adverse outcomes for the mother and fetus, particularly in women with severe chronic hypertension (>170/110mmHg). Overall, there is a ~3-fold ↑ in still birth and ~2.5-fold ↑ in having a small-for-gestational-age baby.[1] The risk of developing pre-eclampsia is ↑ by a factor of 10, and is more likely in women with proteinuria in early pregnancy and if they have had previous pre-eclampsia. Chronic hypertension also ↑ the likelihood of developing gestational diabetes.

Treatment

Although there are no placebo-controlled trials available, historic data suggest that treating severe chronic hypertension in pregnancy reduces maternal and fetal risks.[2] Therefore, antihypertensive therapy should be initiated if the BP is >170/110mmHg.

In pregnant women with mild/moderate chronic hypertension there is good evidence that antihypertensives reduce the risk of developing severe hypertension, which is perhaps unsurprising. However, there is no clear evidence that BP reduction reduces the risks of developing pre-eclampsia or improves maternal or fetal outcomes.[3] Current consensus guidance is split between recommend treatment at a level exceeding 160/100mmHg, or above 140/90mmHg. Given the potential concerns about excessive BP reduction and intra-uterine growth retardation (📖 see Pregnancy, p.184), careful consideration of individual cases is required. Lower thresholds may be appropriate for women with other significant risk factors or previous adverse outcomes.

The target BP is less clear but a reasonable guide would be to aim for a pressure of 130–150/80–100mmHg.

References

1. Allen VM, *et al.* (2004). The effect of hypertensive disorders in pregnancy on small for gestational age and stillbirth: a population based study. *BMC Pregnancy Childbirth* **4**:17.
2. Kincaid-Smith P, *et al.* (1966). Prolonged use of methyldopa in severe hypertension in pregnancy. *BMJ* **1**:274–6.
3. Sibai BM, *et al.* (1990). A comparison of no medication versus methyldopa or labetalol in chronic hypertension during pregnancy. *Am J Obstet Gynec* **162**:960–6.

Pregnancy: gestational hypertension

Gestational hypertension (also known as non-proteinuric PIH) is the most common form of hypertension in pregnancy, affecting ~8% of pregnancies. By definition women must have been normotensive up to 20 weeks' gestation and not have significant proteinuria (<1+ on dipstick). There is clearly an overlap with women with chronic hypertension who have simply not been diagnosed, and also with pre-eclampsia. Although the precise aetiology remains unclear, there is evidently a genetic component.

Known risk factors include:

- Nulliparity.
- Obesity.
- Non-smoker.
- Previous hypertension or high normal BP.
- Pre-existing or gestational diabetes.
- Family history of hypertension or hypertension in pregnancy.

Physiologically, gestational hypertension results from a hyperdynamic circulation with a significantly higher cardiac output and lower resistance than in a normal pregnancy. In contrast to women who go on to develop pre-eclampsia, this state remains until term, and does *not* transform into a high resistance state (📖 see Fig. 6.1, p.185).

Risks

Gestational hypertension ↑ the risks of having a small-for-gestational-age new born by 1.5 × the rate in normotensives, but does not seem to ↑ the risk of still birth significantly.[1] Although gestational hypertension is associated with ↑ perinatal mortality this seems largely driven by a reduced birth weight.[2] Recent data indicate that gestational hypertension ↑ the risk of future CV in the mother by ~2-fold.[3]

The risk of gestational hypertension progressing to pre-eclampsia is ~20%. Risk factors for this include early onset of hypertension and previous miscarriage.

Treatment

Severe (>170/110mmHg) gestational hypertension merits antihypertensive therapy. Although treatment of lower levels of BP halves the risk of developing severe hypertension, there is little evidence that it reduces the risk of perinatal death, premature delivery, or intra-uterine growth retardation. Current guidance suggests initiating therapy if the BP is >140–160/90–100mHg. Given the physiological abnormalities underlying this form of hypertension β-blockade may be an appropriate 1st choice. A target BP of 130–140/80–100mmHg would seem appropriate.

References

1. Allen VM, *et al.* (2004). The effect of hypertensive disorders in pregnancy on small for gestational age and stillbirth: a population based study. *BMC Pregnancy Childbirth* **4**:17.
2. Steer PJ, *et al.* (2004). Maternal blood pressure in pregnancy, birth weight, and perinatal mortality in first births: prospective study. *BMJ* **329**:1312.
3. Ray JG, *et al.* (2005). Cardiovascular health after maternal placental syndromes (CHAMPS): population-based retrospective cohort study. *Lancet* **366**:1797–803.

Pregnancy: pre-eclampsia

Pre-eclampsia (also known as PPIH) affects ~3% of pregnancies and carries a considerable burden of maternal and perinatal morbidity and mortality. It ↑ the risk of still birth by a factor of ~2, and of intra-uterine growth retardation by ~3.

Definition

It is often considered as a triad of hypertension, proteinuria, and oedema after 20 weeks. However it is usually defined as new onset hypertension (>140/90mmHg) in the presence of proteinuria (≥+1 on dipstick, or >300mg/24h). Clearly, it may also complicate chronic or gestational hypertension. It is very rare before 24 weeks' gestation.

Pathophysiology

Pre-eclampsia is a multisystem disorder driven by the placenta that remains incompletely understood. Ineffective placentation following abnormal trophoblastic invasion, leads to placental hypoxia, intra-uterine growth retardation, and release of a number of inflammatory and other factors that trigger a cascade of events in the maternal circulation. There is widespread endothelial dysfunction, a reduction in plasma volume and cardiac output, vasoconstriction, and the development of hypertension. There is also ↑ platelet aggregation, intravascular coagulation, and reduced organ perfusion particularly of the kidney, liver, and brain.

The mechanisms underlying defective placentation are complex and probably relate to a maladaptive interaction between maternal and 'foreign' placental antigens. There is clearly a genetic component, but this is by no means absolute. Of recent interest has been ↑ circulating levels of sFlt1 (a soluble secreted ectodomain) in pre-eclamptics, which leads to lower activity of VEGF.

Risk factors

Epidemiological studies have identified a number of risk factors for developing pre-eclampsia[1] including:

- Aged <20 or >35 years.
- Primigravida (relative risk (RR) 3).
- Multipara with new partner.
- Multiple pregnancy (RR for twins 4).
- Obesity (RR 9).
- Chronic hypertension (RR 3).
- Diabetes.
- Hypercholesterolaemia/triglyceridaemia.
- Renal disease.
- Family history of pre-eclampsia.
- Previous pre-eclampsia (risk of recurrence ~12%).
- Thrombophilia.
- Black.

Signs and symptoms

Pre-eclampsia usually presents after 20 weeks, and is cured by delivery of the placenta, but there are rare reports of pre-eclampsia occurring up to 1 month post-partum. There is considerable overlap between pre-eclampsia and the HELLP syndrome (Box 6.1) and disorders such as thrombotic thrombocytopenia and haemolytic-uraemic syndrome. 📖 Features of severe pre-eclampsia are given in Box 6.2.

The classic features of pre-eclampsia may occur rapidly or insidiously over several days. It is important to ensure that BP is assessed and urine dipped in any pregnant woman who is non-specifically unwell.

- Headache, nausea, blurred vision.
- Hypertension.
- Epigastric pain, abdominal tenderness.
- Peripheral oedema.
- Brisk reflexes, clonus.
- Retinal haemorrhages, cotton wool spots, and papilloedema.
- Confusion, seizures (eclampsia).

Box 6.1 HELLP syndrome

HELLP is considered as a variant form of severe pre-eclampsia in which there is marked disseminated intravascular coagulation, micro-angiopathic haemolytic anaemia, and hepatocellular damage. Between 4–12% of women with pre-existing pre-eclampsia may develop superimposed HELLP. It is associated with considerable ↑ risks, including maternal death) and invariably necessitates urgent delivery. It is defined as:

- Haemolysis (red blood cell destruction of film and elevated lactate dehydrogenase).
- Elevated Liver enzymes (aspartate aminotranferase (AST), alanine aminotransferase (ALT)).
- Low Platelets (<150 × 10^9/L).

Investigations

- FBC ± clotting.
- Uric acid—a sensitive marker of the severity of pre-eclampsia.
- U&Es, creatinine.
- LFTs.
- Urine dipstick, midstream urine.
- Consider urinary VMA, and abdominal USS.

Doppler ultrasound of uterine artery blood flow demonstrates characteristic abnormalities in women with pre-eclampsia (📖 Fig. 6.4), particularly in the mid-trimester. It can also be used early in pregnancy to identify women at ↑ risk of developing pre-eclampsia.[2] Accuracy may be improved when combined with serum markers e.g. PP-13. This is of particular benefit in those deemed to be at ↑ risk by virtue of known risk factors.

Prevention

A number of studies have assessed the impact of a range of preventive treatments including low dose aspirin, antioxidants, and calcium. These have mostly been negative (except calcium supplementation if low calcium intake), and routine administration of these agents, even in women identified at risk of pre-eclampsia, is not currently recommended.

Management

Hospitalization should be considered for women with any of the following adverse features (women without such features may be considered for management at home with frequent (weekly) outpatient review. *Do not forget* extra scans for fetal well-being if there are signs of placental insufficiency as the fetal condition may deteriorate rapidly if pre-eclampsia worsens):

- Clinical feature such as headache, abdominal pain
- BP >140/90mmHg.
- Proteinuria >+1.
- Hyperuricaemia.
- Platelet count $<100 \times 10^9$/L.
- Oligohydramnios or inadequate fetal growth.

Management in hospital will depend on the severity of the disease, gestational age, and response to therapy. Delivery is the only 'cure' for pre-eclampsia but may be delayed if gestation is <34 weeks and there is a good clinical response to therapy and few other adverse signs. Nevertheless, close monitoring of clinical, biochemical, and fetal parameters is essential. Steroids may also be useful in accelerating fetal lung maturation if <34 weeks. It is important to involve a multidisciplinary team at an early stage and management should be carried out in a specialist area.

General management includes regular observations, urine output and analysis, and bed rest. Excessive fluid replacement should be avoided as this has been associated with an ↑ risk of death. Urine outputs as low as 10mL/h may be acceptable. Thromboprophylaxis with thromboembolic deterrent (TED) stockings and low-molecular-weight heparin should be undertaken.

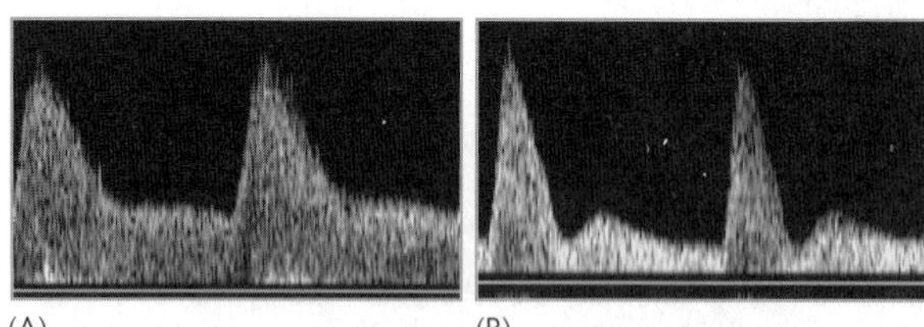

(A) (B)

Fig. 6.4 Doppler flow velocity waveforms in the uterine artery. (A) normal; (B) pre-eclampsia. (Courtesy of Dr Christoph Lees, Cambridge.)

Box 6.2 Severe pre-eclampsia

Defined as 1 or more of the following:

- Severe nausea and vomiting, headache, visual disturbance, abdominal or chest pain, dyspnoea.
- BP >160/110mmHg, oliguria, pulmonary oedema, abruption placentae.
- Platelets <100 × 10^9/L, elevated liver enzymes, albumin <18g/L, heavy proteinuria.

The onset of eclampsia is more likely if there is severe headache, brisk reflexes or clonus, visual disturbances.

Pharmacological treatment

The main aim should be to reduce maternal BP slowly to <160/110mmHg. There is no evidence that tighter control to <140/90mmHg results in better outcomes and it may adversely affect placental perfusion and foetal growth.

Severe hypertension

Depending upon the clinical situation, this may necessitate the use of IV therapy with Labetalol or hydralazine.[3] There is little difference between the 2, although meta-analysis suggests that hydralazine may be associated with more maternal side effects but less foetal bradycardia.[4] Attempts to reduce BP with oral short-acting nifedipine or labetolol may cause uncontrolled reductions in BP and are probably best avoided. Typical regimens are:

- Labetalol slow bolus of 20–40mg, followed by an infusion of 20mg/h max 160mg/h.
- Hydralazine 200–300mcg/min initially then 50–150mcg/min maintenance.

Mild–moderate hypertension

The aim should be to reduce the BP slowly using oral therapy to a target of 140–160/80–100mmHg. Suitable agents include methyldopa, Labetalol, or nifedipine. ACEIs and ARAs should be avoided.

Magnesium sulphate

The MAGPIE Study demonstrated that women with severe pre-eclampsia should receive $MgSO_4$ to terminate and prevent seizures. This is usually given as 4g over 5–15min followed by an infusion of 1g/h.

Follow up

It is important to remember that maximum BP levels are achieved 3–5 days postpartum. Adequate follow-up must be arranged (e.g. 1 week after discharge). The decision concerning if, and when, to discontinue antihypertensives will depend on a number of factors including severity of BP elevation, pre-existing hypertension, and current BP. However, women who have experienced pre-eclampsia are at ↑ risk of developing both hypertension and CVD (📖 Fig. 6.5).

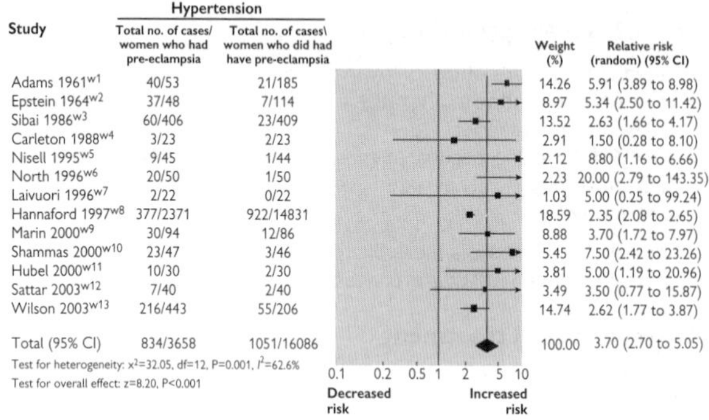

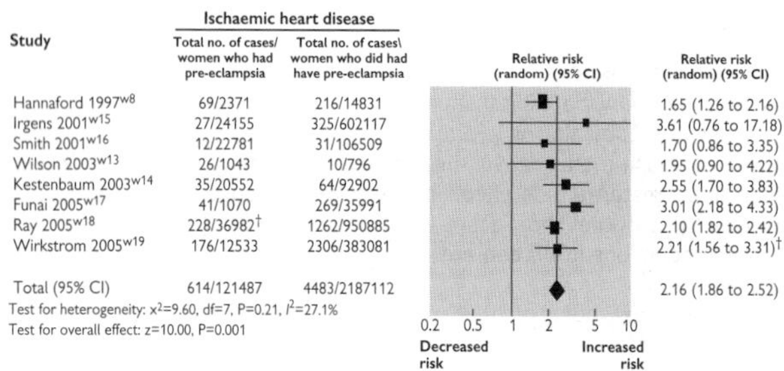

Fig. 6.5 Risk of developing hypertension (top) of ischaemic heart disease (bottom) in women with previous pre-eclampsia. Reproduced from Bellamy L, *et al.* (2007). Pre-eclampsia and risk of cardiovascular disease and cancer in later life: systematic review and meta-analysis *BMJ* **335**: 974, with permission from the BMJ Publishing Group.

References

1. Magnussen EB, *et al.* (2007). Prepregnancy cardiovascular risk factors as predictors of pre-eclampsia: population based cohort study. *BMJ* **355**:978
2. Papageorghiou AT, *et al.* (2001). Multicenter screening for pre-eclampsia and fetal growth restriction by transvaginal uterine artery Doppler at 23 weeks of gestation. *Ultrasound Obstet Gynecol* **18**:441–9.
3. von Dadelszen P, *et al.* (2007). Evidence-based management for preeclampsia. *Front Biosci* **12**:2876–89.
4. Magee LA, *et al.* (2003). Hydralazine for treatment of severe hypertension in pregnancy: meta-analysis. *BMJ* **327**:955.

Diabetes

Diabetes and hypertension frequently co-exist: ~20% of those with type-1 and ~80% of those with type-2 diabetes are hypertensive. Subjects with hypertension are also more likely to develop diabetes than normotensive individuals. In type-2 diabetics there is often clustering of hypertension with other components of the metabolic syndrome such as insulin resistance, obesity, and low HDL-cholesterol. ~85% of the excess CV risk observed in diabetes may be attributed to hypertension.

Pathophysiology of hypertension

Early abnormalities in diabetics include ↑ cardiac output and centralization of venous blood volume. This is accompanied by a loss of the normal night-time BP 'dipping' which is a prelude to the development of albuminuria and LVH. Once established, diabetic hypertension is often 'salt-sensitive', with a corresponding low plasma renin. Diabetes also exaggerates the age-related ↑ in BP, and thus diabetics tend to develop ISH at an earlier age (📖 Fig. 6.6). Postural hypothension is also more common in diabetics due to autonomic failure which can make treating supine hypertension difficult.

The kidney

The presence of micro- (or macro-) albuminuria substantially ↑ CV risk in diabetics. The precise relationship between renal failure, hypertension, and diabetes is unclear but in type 1 diabetes hypertension is probably more a consequence of renal impairment, than a cause. Nevertheless, aggressive BP control reduces the rate of renal decline and also the degree of proteinuria. Blockade of the renin–angiotensin system may also have direct BP-independent reno-protective effects (📖 Figs 6.7 and 6.8). Non-dihydropyridine (DHP) CCAs may also be reno-protective (📖 see Calcium-channel antagonists, p.218).

Treatment

Multiple risk factor intervention is required in diabetics, particularly because of the clustering of risk factors in type-2 patients. A number of randomized controlled trials, such as HOT, UKPDS, and ABCD, have confirmed the efficacy of BP lowering in hypertensive diabetics, including those with ISH (SHEP and SystEur). They also confirm that greater BP reduction yields additional benefits. Consequently, the BHS and JNC-7 target for diabetics is 130/80, which will require combination therapy for most patients.

The relative merits of different antihypertensives in diabetics have been hotly debated, and contradictory evidence has emerged from a number of largely underpowered studies such as UKPDS, CAPP, and ABCD. However, ALLHAT included 13,101 diabetics and 1399 subjects with impaired fasting glucose, and found no difference in outcomes between an ACEI, DHPs, or thiazides (📖 Fig. 6.9). Nevertheless, most authorities recommend that initial therapy in diabetes includes an ACEI or ARA due to their reno-protective effects.

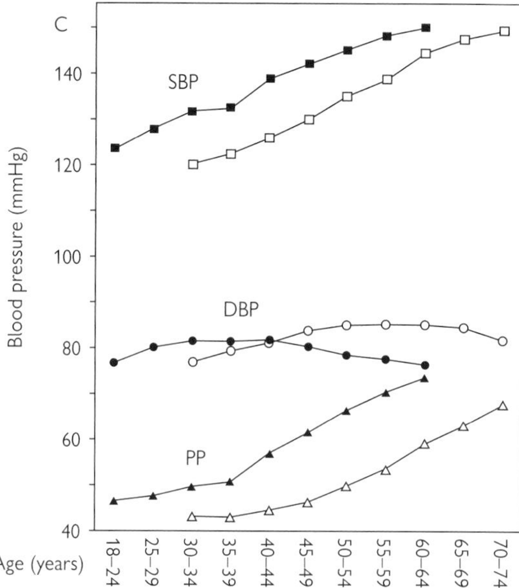

Fig. 6.6 Age-related changes in BP for diabetics (filled symbols) and non-diabetics (open symbols). Redrawn with permission from Rönnback M, *et al.* (2004). Altered age-related blood pressure pattern in type. *Circulation* **110**:1076–82.

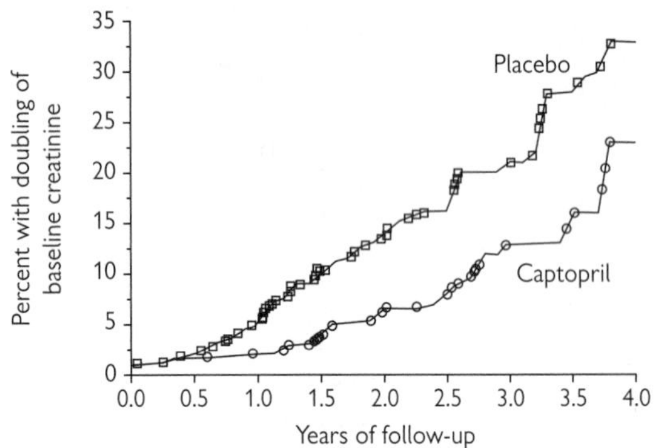

Fig. 6.7 Effect of ACEI on progression of renal dysfunction in patients with insulin-dependent diabetes. Redrawn with permission from Lewis EJ, *et al.* (1993). The effect of angiotensin-converting-enzyme inhibition on diabetic nephropathy. *NEJM* **329**:1456–62.

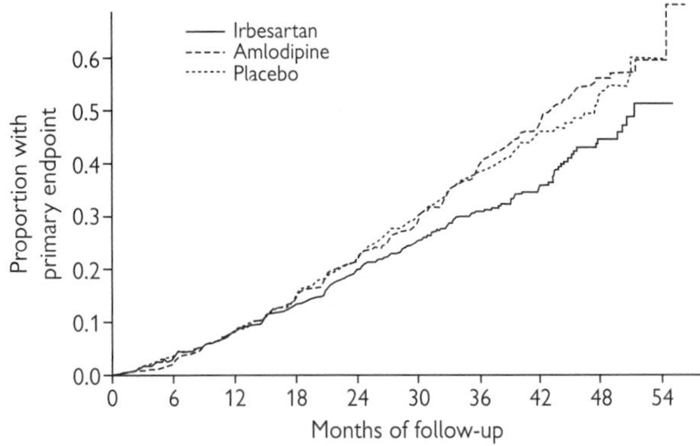

Fig. 6.8 Effect of an ARA compared to placebo or a DHP CCA (control for ↓ BP) on progression of renal dysfunction in patients with type-2 diabetes. Redrawn with permission from Lewis EJ, *et al.* (2001). Renoprotective effect of the angiotensin-receptor antagonist irbesartan in patients with nephropathy due to type 2 diabetes. *NEJM* **345**:851–60.

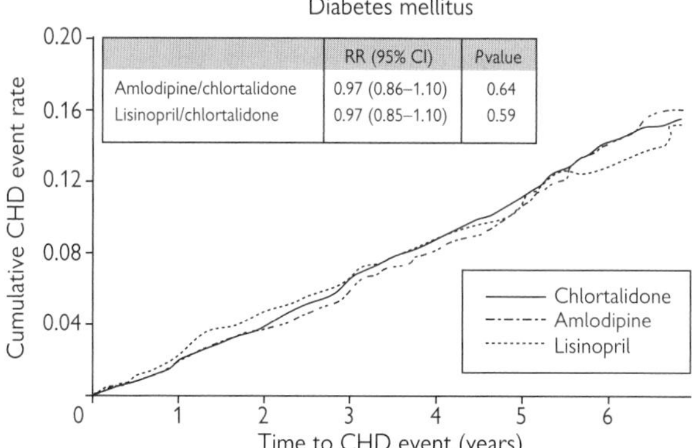

Fig. 6.9 CHD events for the three treatment groups in ALLHAT. Redrawn with permission from Whelton PK, *et al.* (2005). Clinical outcomes in antihypertensive treatment of type 2 diabetes, impaired fasting glucose concentration, and normoglycemia: antihypertensive and lipid-lowering treatment to prevent heart attack trial (ALLHAT). *Arch Intern Med* **165**:1401–9.

The elderly

The prevalence of hypertension ↑ dramatically with age. The recent Health Survey for England[1] reported that ~60% of 60–70-year-olds, and ~80% of those >80 years are hypertensive. The most common form of hypertension in the >60s is ISH, which outnumbers SDH and IDH by ~2:1. ISH is largely a consequence of arterial stiffening, and only a minority of patients seem to progress from SDH or IDH to ISH.

BP and risk

Although SBP and DBP both predict CV risk in older individuals, SBP is more strongly related to risk. Moreover, for a given level of SBP, DBP is inversely related to risk. Hence, pulse pressure (SBP – DBP) is the best predictor of risk in elderly subjects. Nevertheless, because most guidelines and therapeutic trials are based on systolic and diastolic pressure, systolic pressure should be the 1° target in older subjects.

Risks

The proportional risk of MI and stroke associated with a given difference in BP is greater in middle-aged than older subjects by a factor of 2. However, the absolute risks are greater in older subjects due to the substantially higher risk of CVD.

Treatment

Lifestyle modification

Non-pharmacological intervention is effective in older hypertensives. The TONE study[2] demonstrated that salt restriction and weight reduction in the elderly both significantly reduce BP in elderly subjects, particularly when combined (📖 Table 6.1). Older subjects should also be encouraged to ↓ alcohol intake and take regular exercise.

Pharmacological therapy

A number of placebo controlled trials including the EWPHE, MRC-Elderly, and STOP have clearly demonstrated that BP reduction reduces CV events in elderly subjects (📖 Fig. 6.10). The relative reduction in MI and stroke is similar to that seen in middle-aged subjects (33 and 20% respectively). SHEP, SystEur, and SystChina have also confirmed the benefits of treated systolic hypertension in elderly subjects (📖 see Table 2.1, p.54).

Side-effects

Overall, adverse events seem no more common in elderly subjects than in younger subjects, and concerns relating to dizziness and postural hypotension seem largely unjustified. In the SHEP pilot study and STOP trial discontinuation rates were similar between the placebo and active therapy groups.

Choice of agent

Although STOP-2 suggested that there were no differences in outcome between old and newer antihypertensive drugs, the MRC-Elderly Study and a subgroup analysis of the LIFE trial cast doubt on the benefit of β-blockade in older subjects. This was supported by a meta-analysis of trials involving β-blockers or diuretics in elderly hypertensives.[3] Based on the available evidence and the observation that elderly hypertensive subjects usually have a low plasma renin, it seems logical to initiate therapy with a thiazide diuretic or CCA. ACEI and ARAs may also be appropriate 1st-line therapy and are often used to good effect in combination with a diuretic or CCA. Potent vasodilators may precipitate syncope or breathlessness in older subjects particularly in those with systolic hypertension which may relate to the lowering of diastolic pressure and myocardial ischaemia. Nitrates may prove useful in some resistant patients (see Nitrates, p.237).

Table 6.1 Changes in BP in the Tone study[2]

Intervention	Change in BP (systolic/diastolic: mean ± SEM)
Sodium reduction	–3.4 ± 0.8/–1.9 ± 0.5
Weight loss	–4.0 ± 1.3/–1.1 ± 0.8
Combined intervention	–5.3 ± 1.1/–0.34 ± 0.6
Control group	–0.8 ± 0.8/–0.8 ± 0.5

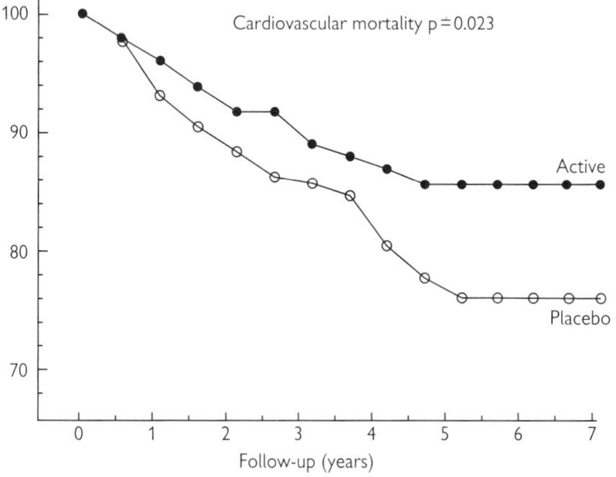

Fig. 6.10 Results of the EWPHE study of hydrochlorothiazide/triamterene versus placebo in elderly patients. Redrawn from Amery A, *et al.* (1985). Mortality and morbidity results from the European Working Party on High Blood Pressure in the Elderly trial. 6105 individuals with previous stroke or transient ischaemic attack. *Lancet* **1**:1349–54, ©1985, with permission from Elsevier.

Targets

JNC 7 recommends a target of <140/90 and the BHS <140/85mmHg. However, the systolic target is often difficult to achieve in elderly subjects and particularly those with ISH.[4] Nevertheless, placebo controlled trials indicate that modest (10/5) reductions in BP produce substantial ↓ in events (↓ CV events by 1/3rd).

Although epidemiological data have consistently disproved the existence of a J-shape curve at least down to 115/75mmHg, a retrospective analysis of the SHEP study[5] suggested that lowering DBP to <70mmHg was associated with an ↑ risk of events (📖 Fig. 6.11). Practically, one should be cautious in producing excessive falls in DBP in older subjects with systolic hypertension, accepting that this may leave imperfect control of SBP.

The very elderly

Few data exist regarding the benefits of BP reduction in the very elderly (>80 years) with ISH. A recent meta-analysis of ~1600 patients >80 years of age[6] demonstrated significant reductions in the incidence of stroke and heart failure with antihypertensive therapy, but no reduction in mortality. The recently published HYVET trial confirmed the substantial benefits of BP ↓ in older subjects.

References

1. Primatesta P and Poulter NR (2006). Improvement in hypertension management in England: results from the Survey for England 2003. *J Hypertens* **24**:1187–92.
2. Stamler R, *et al.* (1987). Nutritional therapy for high blood pressure. Final report of a four-year randomized controlled trial – the Hypertension Control Program. *JAMA* **257**:1484–8.
3. Messerli FH, *et al.* (1998). Are beta-blockers efficacious as first-line therapy for hypertension in the elderly? A systematic review. *JAMA* **279**:1903–7.
4. Mancia G and Grassi G (2002). Systolic and diastolic blood pressure control in antihypertensive drug trials. *J Hypertension* **20**:1461–4.
5. Somes GW, *et al.* (1999). The role of diastolic blood pressure when treating isolated systolic hypertension. *Arch Intern Med* **159**:2004–9.
6. Gueyffier F, *et al.* (1999). Antihypertensive drugs in very old people: a subgroup meta-analysis of randomised controlled trials. INDIANA Group. *Lancet* **353**:793–6.

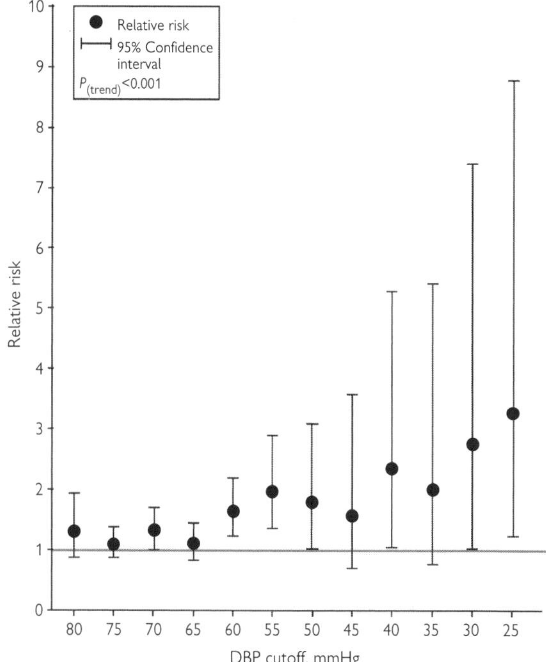

Fig. 6.11 Relationship between achieve diastolic pressure and relative risk of CV disease in the SHEP study. Reproduced with permission from Somes GW, *et al.* (1999). The role of diastolic blood pressure when treating isolated systolic hypertension. *Arch Intern Med* **159**: 2004–9.

Children

BP in children is considerably lower than in adults, and ↑ steadily throughout childhood (📖 Fig. 6.12). Systolic and diastolic pressures ↑ more steeply in puberty, particularly in boys, and are positively related to weight and inversely to height. There is also considerable (although not complete) tracking of BP throughout childhood and into adult life. Hypertension in children is rare and should prompt a thorough search for 2° causes, especially if the child is not overweight.

Definitions

Defining hypertension in children is even more problematic than in adults, due to the variability in BP, the clear age-dependency, and the lack of outcome data. While the 'usual' adult definition of 140/90mmHg can be applied, the standard approach is to use age-related percentile data as a reference (📖 Fig. 6.12). Hypertension is usually defined as a pressure consistently above the 98th centile for age and 'high normal pressure' if consistently between the 90–95th centiles. However, as is apparent for the centile graph, after the age of 16 years the 95th centile for systolic pressure approximates to a value of 140mmHg, suggesting that the 140/90 cut-off may be more appropriate after this age.

Prevalence of hypertension

Using the 98th age-related centile as a cut-off, the estimated prevalence of hypertension in children is ~2%, and ~7% are classified as 'high normal BP.[1] The predominant form of hypertension is ISH and is physiologically driven largely by an ↑ cardiac output and, to a lesser extent, stiffening of the large arteries.[2] Mixed systolic/diastolic and diastolic are relatively rare, and more suggestive of an underlying cause.

BP measurement

The most important aspect is to select an appropriately-sized cuff, rather than rely on the standard adult cuff (80–100% of the arm circumference)—too small a cuff will lead to an over estimation of BP. Systolic pressure is taken as Korotkoff I and diastolic as V (not IV). Oscillometric devices may be used, but most are rarely validated in children. The role of ABPM in children is unclear and it is not recommended as a standard part of the clinical assessment at present.

Aetiology

The vast majority of childhood hypertension is essential. The main risk factors for essential hypertension in childhood appear to be weight, obesity (weight adjusted for height), and family history. There is little influence of gender and race. Recent data from the USA suggest that the rate of hypertension amongst children is rising in parallel with the ↑ levels of obesity. Although relatively rare, 2° hypertension is the predominant form of hypertension in younger children. The most frequent underlying cause is renal parenchymal disease (📖 Table 6.2).

Table 6.2 Causes of hypertension by age group.

Pre-puberty	Pubertal-adolescence
Renal parenchymal disease	Essential hypertension
Renovascular disease	General illness
Endocrine causes	Renal parenchymal disease
Co-arctation	Renovascular disease
Essential hypertension	Endocrine causes
	Co-arctation
	Drugs e.g. contraceptive pill

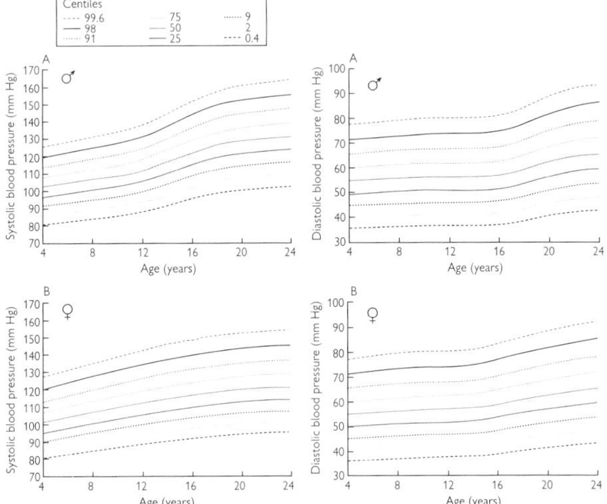

Fig. 6.12 BP centiles for children in the UK. Reproduced from Jackson LV, *et al.* (2007). Blood pressure centiles for Great Britain. *Arch Dis Child* **92**:298–303, with permission from the BMJ Publishing Group.

Investigations

The precise investigation will depend on the severity of the hypertension, clues to a possible underlying cause (📖 Table 6.3), and the results of screening tests. All patients need a thorough examination and fundoscopy.

Screening/general
- FBC, ESR.
- U&Es, Ca^{2+}, CRP, TSH.
- Renal ultrasound.
- Urine analysis.
- ECG.

Specific
- Urinary VMA/catecholamines.
- Renin/aldosterone.
- Echo.
- MR-angiogram.
- Isotope renal scan.

Treatment

For those with essential hypertension, targeted lifestyle intervention can be of considerable benefit especially for those with borderline or mildly elevated BP. This includes weight control, regular exercise, a reduction in salt intake, and ↑ in fruit and vegetables in the diet. Obvious precipitants such as the contraceptive pill and illicit drugs should be stopped.

Pharmacological therapy may be required if lifestyle changes fail, or in more severe cases of hypertension. Unfortunately, in the UK most antihypertensives are not licensed for use in children, and relatively few data concerning efficacy and side effects are available. However, the Food and Drug Administration Modernization Act in the USA has led to a number of studies of new antihypertensive agents in children being performed. Nevertheless, most recommendations are extrapolation of observations in adults and previous clinical experience.

The initial choice of therapy should be based on experience, and documented safety and efficacy. Evidence of efficacy in children is now available for the 4 main classes of antihypertensive drug, and all should be considered as suitable initial therapy. Comorbidities may be a compelling indication for use of a particular class of drug e.g. diabetic nephropathy and ACEi, or co-arctation and a β-blocker. The underlying pathophysiology, e.g. raised renin, may also help in the initial choice of drug. Suggested doses and indications are listed in 📖 Table 6.4. Some agents are also available as suspensions which aid accurate dosing, but this is usually as 'specials' and not 'off the shelf'.

Table 6.3 Features suggestive of 2° hypertension

Cause	Features
Phaeochromocytoma	Sweating, tachycardia, flushing
Co-arctation	Murmur
Renal artery stenosis	Abdo bruit, ↑ creatinine on ACEI, ↑ renal mass, active urinary sediment
Endocrine cause	Acne, hirsutism, muscle weakness, obesity, ↓ K^+
Vasculitis	Rash, joint pain swelling, ↑ ESR/CRP, active urinary sediment

Table 6.4 Examples of drugs which may be used in the management of hypertension in children

Class	Examples	Dose*
Diuretics	Bendroflumethiazide	50–100mcg/kg OD; 12–18 years 2.5–5mg
β-blockers	Atenolol	0.5–2mg/kg OD; 12–18 years 50mg OD
	Propranolol	0.25–1mg/kg TDS; 12–18 years 80mg BD initially
ACEIs	Lisinopril	70mcg/kg OD; 12–18 years 2.5–20mg OD
AT1 receptor antagonists	Losartan	20–50kg 25mg OD; ≥50kg 50mg OD
CCAs	Amlodipine	100–400mcg/kg OD; 12–18 years 5–10mg OD

*Dose assumes age <12 years, unless otherwise stated. Always check the dose in the British National Formulary for Children. None of the drugs are licensed for use in children and should be used under specialist care only.

References

1. Jackson LV, *et al.* (2007). Blood pressure centiles for Great Britain. *Arch Dis Child* **92**:298–303.
2. McEniery CM, *et al.* (2005). Increased stroke volume and aortic stiffness contribute to isolated systolic hypertension in young adults. *Hypertension* **46**:221–6.

Post-stroke

Hypertension is the most potent risk factor for ischaemia and haemorrhagic stroke, and the role of BP reduction in the 1° prevention of stroke is firmly established. Recent studies have also demonstrated the role of BP lowering in 2° prevention. However, the management of hypertension in the acute setting remains controversial.

Acute stroke

The majority of individuals who survive the immediate event will be hypertensive, due in part to pre-existing hypertension but also the acute pressor effects of cerebral ischaemia, hypoxia, pain, etc. Physiologically, raised BP may help to ↑ perfusion in the area surrounding the area of ischaemic necrosis (the penumbra), thus limiting the extent of neurological damage. Conversely, an excessive rise in BP may ↑ the risk of haemorrhagic transformation following cerebral infarction, or lead to an extension of a haemorrhagic event. It is these 2 opposing views that have led to considerable variation in the BP management following an acute stroke. Studies, including CHIPS, are ongoing and will address the impact of BP lowing but at present most of the guidance is based on consensus opinion.

Mild or moderate hypertension (~200/120mmHg) in the context of an acute cerebral event probably requires no medical intervention. Aggressive sudden BP reduction may lead to an extension of cerebral injury and is probably best avoided. However, pre-existing antihypertensive medication is probably best continued (assuming previous compliance with medication is likely). Slow acting oral antihypertensive therapy may be initiated after the initial 24–48 h.

Severe hypertension is more controversial. Although there is no hard evidence either way, cautious reduction of BP with IV agents may be justified especially in the context of a haemorrhagic stroke and a DBP >120mmHg. For ischaemic events a higher cut-off of 220/130mmHg may be appropriate. Whatever the decision, controlled cautious BP reduction is probably safest, and rapid drops in BP using sodium nitroprusside should be avoided.

2° prophylaxis

Lowering BP to prevent recurrent strokes would seem a logical intervention based on epidemiological data and a meta-analysis of small intervention trials would support this view.[1] The PATS study confirmed the efficacy of the thiazide diuretic indapamide in this situation, and the PROGRESS Study demonstrated a significant reduction in recurrent stroke for the combination of ACEI and thiazide but not ACEI alone (📖 Fig. 6.13). Based on these data, and the fact that most stroke patients are elderly and tend to have low plasma renin, a thiazide would seem a sensible initial choice for BP reduction, although co-existing conditions such as diabetes should also be taken into consideration. A target pressure of 130/80 post-stroke is recommended by the BHS.

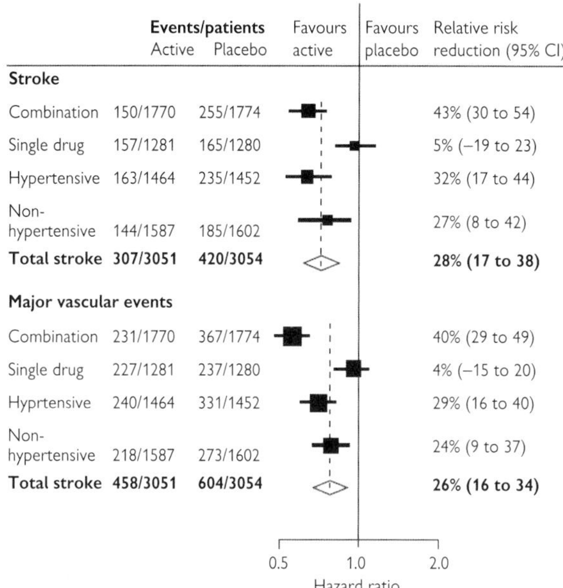

Events/patients
Active Placebo
Favours active
Favours placebo
Relative risk reduction (95% CI)
Stroke
Combination 150/1770 255/1774 43% (30 to 54)
Single drug 157/1281 165/1280 5% (−19 to 23)
Hypertensive 163/1464 235/1452 32% (17 to 44)
Non-hypertensive 144/1587 185/1602 27% (8 to 42)
Total stroke 307/3051 420/3054 28% (17 to 38)
Major vascular events
Combination 231/1770 367/1774 40% (29 to 49)
Single drug 227/1281 237/1280 4% (−15 to 20)
Hyprtensive 240/1464 331/1452 29% (16 to 40)
Non-hypertensive 218/1587 273/1602 24% (9 to 37)
Total stroke 458/3051 604/3054 26% (16 to 34)
0.5
1.0
2.0
Hazard ratio

Fig. 6.13 Results of the PROGRESS study examining the effect of placebo, perindopril or the combination of indapamide and perindopril post stroke. Reproduced from PROGRESS Collaborative Group (2001). Randomised trial of a perindopril-based blood-pressure-lowering regimen among 6105 individuals with previous stroke or transient ischaemic attack. *Lancet* **358**: 1033–41, © 2001, with permission from Elsevier.

Reference

1. Rodgers A, *et al.* (1997). The effects of blood pressure lowering in individuals with cerebrovascular disease: an overview of randomised controlled trials. *Neurol Rev Int* **2**:12–15

Transplant patients

Hypertension post-transplantation is common, affecting up to 80% of organ recipients, and is an important cause of excess morbidity and mortality. The long-term survival of renal grafts is dependent on post-transplant BP, which also predicts the risk of acute rejection. Hypertension also ↑ the likelihood of allograft vasculopathy and the development of diffuse coronary atherosclerosis in cardiac transplants.

A number of mechanisms are responsible for post-transplant hypertension, including pre-existing hypertension, CVD, impaired kidney function, and the use of immunosuppressants including calcineurin inhibitors and corticosteroids. Hypertension appears to be more common with ciclosporine than with tacrolimus but this may relate to differences in potency and concomitant steroid use.

Physiologically, early post-transplant hypertension is often related to a hyperdynamic circulation and salt and water retention. This usually translates into an ↑ peripheral resistance and return of cardiac output to normal. Calcineurin inhibitors have also been associated with impaired endothelial function and activation of the sympathetic nervous system.

Treatment

There are no large RCTs comparing the efficacy of different classes of anti-hypertensive agents in the post-transplant situation. DHP CCAs are often favoured in this setting because they reverse the peripheral vasoconstriction associated with calcineurin inhibitors. Some inhibit the metabolism of specific calcineurin inhibitors and, therefore, monitoring plasma levels of the inhibitor may be required.

ACEIs and ARAs tend to be less effective in reducing BP, when used alone, but are more effective when combined with a thiazide diuretic. They also reduce the degree of proteinuria in renal transplant patients, independently of BP, suggesting that they may have additional benefits in this group of patients. However, whether such effects will translate into longer graft survival needs to be formally assessed. It is particularly important to monitor plasma K^+ and creatinine in transplant patients following blockade of the renin–angiotensin system.

β-blockers and thiazide diuretic may also be used, and the former may be particularly useful post-cardiac transplantation, or in patients with established CVD.

No specific targets are set in the post-transplant situation, but it would seem prudent to aim for a lower target of 130/80mmHg in subjects with manifest CVD or diabetes, and following renal transplantation.

Chapter 7

Antihypertensive drugs

Angiotensin-converting enzyme inhibitors

Agents

The first ACEI, captopril, was introduced in 1981. Currently, 11 agents are licensed in the UK and most are available in generic form. ACEIs are a chemically heterogeneous group, but this seems to make little difference to their clinical effects. All except captopril and lisinopril, are pro-drugs that require enzymatic conversion in the liver. Usual starting dose is the equivalent of 5–10mg of lisinopril OD (max dose 40mg): check U&Es after 7–10 days.

Mechanism of action

ACEIs inhibit ACE which catalyses the conversion of the inactive decapeptide angiotensin I to the active octapeptide angiotensin II, and also the breakdown of bradykinin (see Fig. 1.11 p.17). Angiotensin II is a powerful vasoconstrictor and also promotes aldosterone synthesis, sympathetic activity, thirst, and has effects on cell growth and differentiation. Bradykinin is a vasodilating peptide, and ↑ levels contribute to the antihypertensive effect of ACEIs. In hypertension, ACE inhibition produces a balanced reduction of both cardiac pre-load and after-load, through direct and indirect arteriolar dilatation. ACEIs also blunt stress-induced ↑ in catecholamines via their sympatholytic effects, and thus heart rate changes with ACE inhibition are not significant.

Evidence base

There are no large RCTs comparing ACE inhibition to placebo in patients with hypertension, but BP comparator studies indicate that ACEIs are as effective as other drugs. In general ACEIs are less effective in certain sub-groups, including low-renin, salt-sensitive individuals such as older people and blacks. The largest hypertension trial to date, ALLHAT, did not show any difference in the 1° outcome (MI) between lisinopril and chlortalidone or amlodipine (Fig. 7.1). However, lisinopril was slightly less effective in preventing stroke and total CVD (2° outcomes) than the diuretic. Data from several placebo-controlled studies indicate that ACEIs should be used in patients with any degree of heart failure (e.g. SOLVD), and post-MI (AIRE, ISIS). ACEI also reduce the rate of proteinuria, and renal decline in diabetic and non-diabetic subjects with renal impairment independently of BP reduction (REIN). Recent evidence form ASCOT and other studies also suggests that ACEIs may reduce the rate of new-onset diabetes (see Fig. 7.7).

Indications

ACEIs are thought to be more effective at BP reduction in younger subjects due to the higher levels of circulating renin, and relatively less effective in older hypertensives and blacks. However, they are commonly used across all ages of patients.

Compelling indications

- Heart failure.
- Nephropathy.
- Diabetes or insulin resistance.
- Co-existing CVD, especially MI.

Contra-indications

- Pregnancy: associated with pulmonary hypoplasia, fetal skull hypoplasia, growth retardation and renal failure in the fetus.
- Hypersensitivity to ACEIs: including angio-oedema.
- RAS: may be used with expert advice in unilateral disease.

Side effects

- Cough: common up to 10%; a class effect.
- Renal impairment: ► always check U&Es 7–10 days after initiating an ACEI. A limited ↑ in serum creatinine of up to 25% is acceptable, unless hyperkalaemia develops. Monitor electrolytes at regular intervals if any significant rise occurs.
- Hypotension: 1st dose hypotension is rare unless on large doses of diuretics or concomitant heart failure.
- Angio-oedema: <0.1%, but potentially life threatening. Onset may be delayed.
- Rash, loss of taste, GI disturbance, altered LFTs.

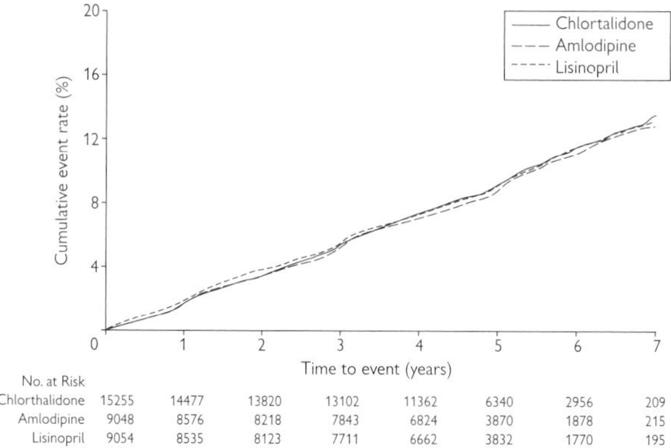

No. at Risk								
Chlorthalidone	15255	14477	13820	13102	11362	6340	2956	209
Amlodipine	9048	8576	8218	7843	6824	3870	1878	215
Lisinopril	9054	8535	8123	7711	6662	3832	1770	195

Fig. 7.1 The ALLHAT study demonstrated no difference between an ACEI, diuretic and CCA for the 1° outcome of MI. Redrawn from The ALLHAT Officers and Coordinators for the ALLHAT Collaborative Research Group (2002). Major outcomes in high-risk hypertensive patients randomized to angiotensin-converting enzyme inhibitor or calcium channel blocker vs diuretic: The Antihypertensive and Lipid-Lowering Treatment to Prevent Heart Attack Trial (ALLHAT). *JAMA* **288**:2981–7.

Angiotensin receptor antagonists

Agents

The antihypertensive effect of a peptide-based ARA (saralasin) was 1st described in the 1970s, but the 1st orally available agent (losartan) was not introduced until 1995. 7 agents are licensed in the UK, and they have differing pharmacological properties. Irbesartan and valsartan are competitive antagonists, whereas candestrtan and losartan are effectively irreversible inhibitors. Losartan is a pro-drug and requires metabolism for most of its clinical effect. There are also differences in bio-availability. However, such differences seem to have little effect on clinical efficacy. Most drugs have a relatively shallow dose–response curve, and require little dose-titration. The usual starting dose is the equivalent of 50mg of losartan OD (max dose 100mg): check U&Es after 7–10 days.

Mechanism of action

Angiotensin II acts on 2 subtypes of receptor, the AT1 receptor and the AT2 receptor. Virtually all the biological effects of angiotensin II result from stimulation of the AT1 receptor. By antagonizing this receptor the ARAs or 'sartans' produce vasodilatation, and tend to lower sympathetic activity and aldosterone secretion.

Evidence base

There are no large, RCTs comparing ARAs to placebo in patients with hypertension, but BP comparator studies indicate that ARAs are as effective as other drugs. The LIFE Study compared atenolol and losartan in older high risk hypertensive subjects, and found a clear advantage in those randomized to losartan, despite equivalent BP reduction. In contrast, the VALUE study showed no difference in the 1° endpoint between valstartan and amlodipine (📖 Fig. 7.2). Overall, the superiority of ARAs appears to be limited to comparisons with β-blockers, and ARAs are probably no more effective than other classes of drug if equivalent BP reduction is achieved. Interestingly, in VALUE and LIFE, there were fewer new cases of diabetes in the ARA cohort; suggesting, that like ACEI, ARAs may prevent the development of diabetes (📖 see Fig. 7.5, p.224). ARAs also reduce the rate of proteinuria, and renal decline in diabetic subjects with renal impairment independently of BP reduction (RENAL and IDNT). Data from several studies also support the use of ARAs in patients with heart failure (ELITE and ValHEFT).

Indications

ARAs are probably more effective at BP reduction in younger subjects due to the higher levels of circulating renin, and relatively less effective in blacks. However, they are commonly used across all ages of patients, particularly if intolerant to ACEIs.

Compelling indications

- Heart failure.
- Nephropathy.
- Diabetes or insulin resistance.

Contra-indications

- Pregnancy: associated with pulmonary hypoplasia, fetal skull hypoplasia, growth retardation, and renal failure in the fetus.
- RAS: may be used with expert advice in unilateral disease.

Side effects

Relatively few, generally very well tolerated.

- Hypotension: 1st dose hypotension is rare unless on large doses of diuretics or concomitant heart failure.
- Angio-oedema: <0.01%, but potentially life threatening. Onset may be delayed.
- Renal impairment: ► always check U&Es 7–10 days after initiating an ARA. A limited ↑ in serum creatinine of up to 35% is acceptable, unless hyperkalaemia develops. Monitor electrolytes at regular intervals if any significant rise occurs.

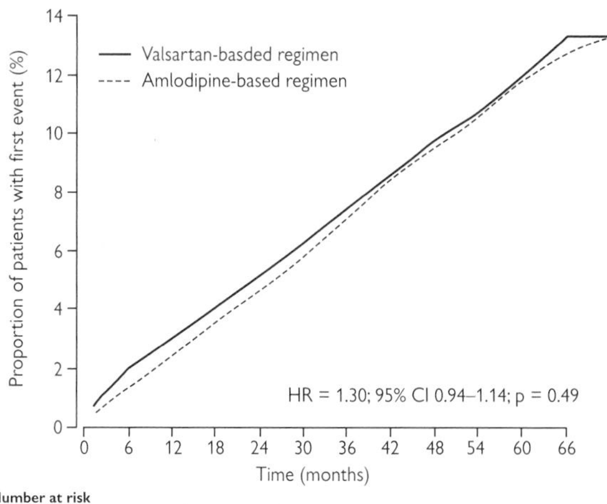

Fig. 7.2 Results from the VALUE study for the primary endpoint of cardiac morbidity and mortality. Redrawn from Julius S *et al.* (2004). Outcomes in hypertensive patients at high cardiovascular risk treated with regimens based on valsartan or amlodipine: the VALUE randomised trial. *Lancet* **363**:2022–31 © 2004, with permission from Elsevier.

Beta-blockers

Agents

β-blockers, first synthesized by James Black in the 1950s (for which he won the Nobel Prize) were introduced into clinical practice in the 1970s. The degree of selectivity for α- versus β-adrenoceptor varies, but with the exception of labetalol and carvediolol, most available agents have little physiological effect on α-adrenoceptors. Propranolol is a non-selective antagonist blocking both β_1 and β_2 adrenocpetors. Most of the other agents in the class are varyingly β_1-selective, nebivolol being the most β_1-selective. Some agents also display intrinsic sympathomimetic activity (e.g. pindolol)—meaning that they are partial agonists at β_1 adrenoceptors. β-blockers also vary considerably in their pharmacokinetics, including $t_{1/2}$ and lipid solubility. Despite the very diverse nature of this class of antihypertensive drug, there are few clinical differences except that β_1-selective and vasodilating agents tend to produce fewer side effects. BP reduction seems comparable. Usual dose range is the equivalent of 2.5–5mg of bisoprolol OD—higher doses are no more effective.

Mechanism of action

Act as antagonists at the β-adrenoceptor, but the mechanism by which this leads to a reduction in BP is unclear. It is likely to be the result of several different effects including a short-term reduction in cardiac output, followed by baro-receptor resetting and effective peripheral vasodilatation. Inhibition of central sympathetic outflow and a reduction in plasma renin levels are also important. Direct vasodilatation may also contribute to BP lowering with drugs that also antagonize α-adrenoceptors, or that display intrinsic sympathomimetic activity, or that release NO (nebivolol).

Evidence base

Many studies have demonstrated comparable BP reduction with β-blockers to other antihypertensive drugs, but despite widespread clinical use there are no RCTs that demonstrate a reduction in mortality with β-blockers compared with placebo. Recently, a number of studies and a meta-analysis (📖 Fig. 7.3) have cast doubt on the efficacy of atenolol in essential hypertension. The MRC-Elderly study found atenolol no better than placebo in older hypertensives, and the more recent LIFE and ASCOT studies suggested that it was inferior to 'newer' agents, despite similar falls in BP. A number of explanations have been offered for this apparent paradox but 2 are favoured. Atenolol, particularly in combination with diuretics seems to ↑ the rate of new-onset diabetes, which may ↑ CV risk and offset the benefits of BP reduction. Alternatively, atenolol seem less effective at reducing central (aortic) BP, despite being equally effective at reducing brachial BP, which may, in part be due to the associated bradycardia (CAFE). Whether we can extrapolate these observations to all β-blockers (particularly the vasodilating ones) is unclear, but based on these data the BHS/NICE guidance has removed them from 1st-line use. However the recent ESH/ESC guidelines have retained them, and they remain useful in young subjects and those with CVD.

Indications

β-blockers may be useful 1st-line in young subjects who are in the hyperkinetic phase of hypertension, and in those with CVD, where they reduce symptoms and may prevent events. They are also indicated in congestive cardiac failure. β-blockers are relatively less effective in older, low-renin subjects and blacks. Despite concerns, β-blockers remain a useful antihypertensive drug and are frequently used in combination with other drugs, although dual therapy with a diuretic is probably best avoided.

Compelling indications

- CVD.
- Dysrhythmias.
- Pregnancy (labetalol).
- Aortic dissection.

Contra-indications

- Asthma: if absolutely required use most β_1-selective agent available.
- Uncontrolled heart failure.
- 2nd- or 3rd-degree heart block.
- RAS: may be used with expert advice in unilateral disease.

Side effects

- Bradycardia, heart failure.
- Bronchospasm.
- Tiredness.
- Cold peripheries.
- Impotence.
- Nightmares.

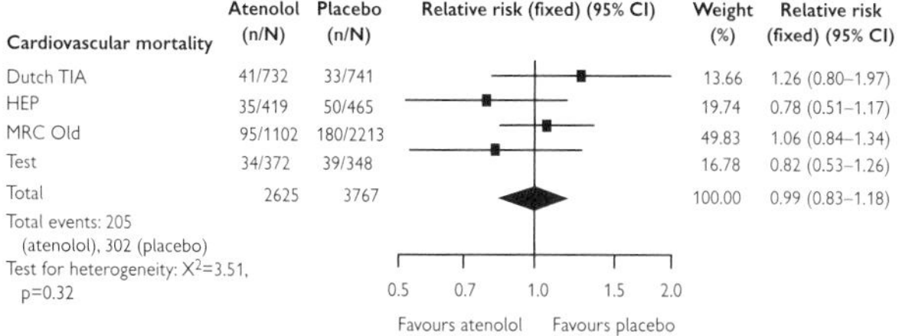

Cardiovascular mortality
Atenolol (n/N)
Placebo (n/N)
Relative risk (fixed) (95% CI)
Weight (%)
Relative risk (fixed) (95% CI)
Dutch TIA 41/732 33/741 13.66 1.26 (0.80–1.97)
HEP 35/419 50/465 19.74 0.78 (0.51–1.17)
MRC Old 95/1102 180/2213 49.83 1.06 (0.84–1.34)
Test 34/372 39/348 16.78 0.82 (0.53–1.26)
Total 2625 3767 100.00 0.99 (0.83–1.18)
Total events: 205 (atenolol), 302 (placebo)
Test for heterogeneity: X2=3.51, p=0.32
0.5 0.7 1.0 1.5 2.0
Favours atenolol
Favours placebo

Fig. 7.3 A meta-analysis of antihypertensive studies involving atenolol. There is no difference between atenolol and placebo in preventing CV mortality (neither was there for total mortality, stroke, nor MI). Redrawn from Carlberg, B, *et al.* (2004). Atenolol in hypertension: is it a wise choice? *Lancet* **365**:1684–9, © 2004 with permission from Elsevier.

Calcium-channel antagonists

Agents

The CCAs are a structurally and pharmacologically diverse group of agents that can be divided into 2 major categories: the dihydropyridine (DHP), and the non-DHPs (the phenylalkylamines and benzothiazepines). There are currently 9 CCAs licensed in the UK, including nifedipine and amlodipine, many of which are available generically. They vary in the pharmacokinetics, particularly $t_{1/2}$, and extended release preparation of some short-acting ones are available (e.g. Adalat-LA®). Only 2 non-DHPs are available: diltiazem and verapamil. Despite the physiological and pharmacological differences BP ↓ seems comparable.

► Usual dose is the equivalent of 5–10 mg of amlodipine OD. Short acting nifedipine should never be used, as it can produce a rapid reduction in BP, leading to stroke, and myocardial ischaemia.

Mechanism of action

All currently available drugs in this class block the L-type calcium channel. The 1° antihypertensive effect results from peripheral vasodilatation due to resistance vessel smooth-muscle relaxation. This is usually associated with a reflex tachycardia and sympathetic activation. In addition, verapamil and diltiazem have negative ionotropic and chronotropic effects (due to blockade of cardiac L-type channels) which leads to fall in cardiac output that contributes to BP ↓.

Evidence base

A number of studies have clearly shown that CCAs have comparable efficacy to other antihypertensive agents (ALLHAT, NORDIL, INSIGHT studies). They have been subject to a placebo-controlled RCT in older subjects with ISH (SystEur) which demonstrated good efficacy—strokes were reduced by ~40% and CV morbidity/mortality by ~30% (Fig. 7.4). Early concerns regarding the safety of CCAs with regard to heart disease, cancer, and bleeding seems unfounded. Although amlodipine was found to be neutral in patients with heart failure (PRAISE), in ALLHAT it was less effective in preventing heart failure than chlortalidone. Thus CCAs should be used with caution in subjects with overt heart failure. The non-DHP agents seem able to reduce proteinuria to a similar degree as ACEIs, but the DHP have no effect. Overall, CCAs seem neutral with regard to the development of new-onset diabetes (📖 see Fig. 7.5).

Indications

CCAs are particularly effective in older subjects, especially those with ISH, and those with low-renin hypertension, such as blacks. The non-DHP CCAs may be useful in patients who need rate control or who have dysrhythmias. CCAs may also be useful in patients with angina, migraine, or Reynaud's phenomenon. Nifedipine is also used in the management of hypertension in pregnancy (unlicensed indication).

Compelling indications

- Reynaud's phenomenon.
- Dysrhythmias (non-DHP).
- Angina.
- Subarachnoid haemorrhage.

Contra-indications

- Severe heart failure.
- Severe aortic stenosis.
- 2nd- or 3rd-degree AV block (non-DHP).

► Take care when combining a non-DHP with a β–blocker as it may precipitate AV block and congestive cardiac failure.

Side effects

- Flushing, headache, ankle swelling—all more common in women.
- Dizziness.
- Palpitations.
- Gum hyperplasia.
- Rash.
- Constipation.

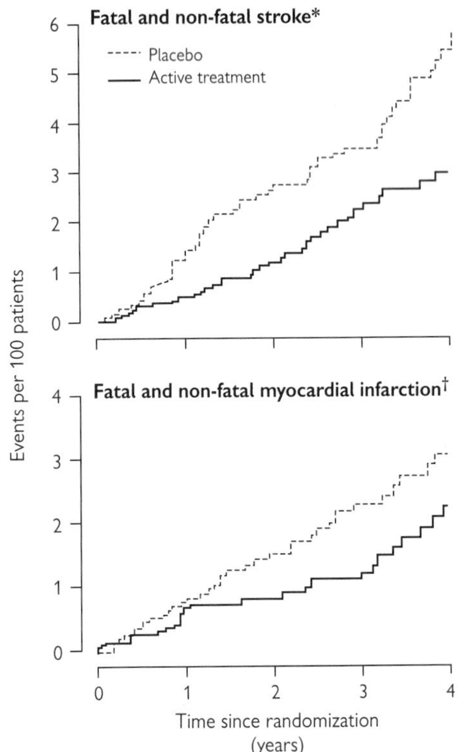

Fig. 7.4 Key results of the SystEur Study a placebo-controlled trial of nitrendipine (a DHP) in ISH. Redrawn from Staessen JA, *et al* (1997). Randomised double-blind comparison of placebo and active treatment for older patients with isolated systolic hypertension. *Lancet* **350**:757–64, © 1997 with permission from Elsevier.

Thiazide diuretics

Agents

Thiazide diuretics were synthesized in the early 1950s, and were the 1st truly effective oral antihypertensive available. 6 thiazide/thiazide-like diuretics are available in the UK, including bendroflumethiazide, indapamide, and chlortalidone (particularly long acting). They are relatively mild diuretics and are used at low doses in hypertension (there is probably a modest dose–response effect). The usual dose range is the equivalent of 2.5–5mg of bendroflumethiazide OD.

Mechanism of action

The exact mechanism of action remains unclear. The acute fall in BP is due to salt and water loss and a reduction in extra-cellular volume. This is a direct result of inhibition of the NCCT in the distal part of the nephron (see Fig. 7.6, p.227). However, with chronic use plasma volume returns to normal and there is a state of peripheral vasodilatation. The mechanism underlying this effect is thought to relate to inhibition of carbonic anhydrase, changes in smooth muscle cell pH, and thus calcium handling. It is not related to inhibition of the NCCT.

Evidence base

Thiazide diuretics were the 1st agents subject to RCTs in hypertension, and they proved effective in reducing stroke and MI (VA trials, Table 7.1). Meta-analysis confirmed this and suggested that low-dose diuretics were more effective than high doses. The ground-breaking SHEP study confirmed the efficacy of thiazides in older subjects with isolated hypertension in a placebo-controlled RCT. The ALLHAT study confirmed the equivalence of thiazides to new drugs (there was actually a greater ↓ in CV events, stroke, and heart failure with chlortalidone than lisinopril). Recently evidence from ASCOT and a subsequent meta-analysis (Fig. 7.5), suggest that long-term therapy with thiazides may significantly ↑ the risk of new-onset diabetes compared to placebo or new agents. However, it is unclear if this is associated with a significant ↑ in CV risk, or whether it is irreversible. Moreover, combination therapy (particularly with an ACEI) may offset this potential risk.

Indications

Thiazides are most effective in older subjects (particularly those with ISH), and in blacks. They work well in combination with ACEIs or ARAs.

Compelling indications

- ISH.
- Blacks.

Contra-indications

- Pregnancy—neonatal thrombocytopenia, oligohydramnios.
- Gout.
- Hypercalcaemia.
- Refractory hypokalaemia or hyponatraemia.

Side effects

- Gout.
- Hypokalaemia/natraemia.
- Postural hypotension.
- Impotence.
- Photosensitivity.

Table 7.1 Results of the VA Co-operative Study which compared hydrochlorothiazide (plus reserpine plus hydralazine) against placebo in subjects with a diastolic pressure of 115–129mmHg.

	Placebo n = 194	Active Rx* n = 186
Accelerated hypertension	4	0
Stroke	20	5
Total coronary event	13	11
Fatal coronary event	11	6
Congestive heart failure	11	0
Renal damage	3	0
Deaths	19	8

Data from Veterans Administration Co-operative Study Group on antihypertensive agents. Effects of treatment on morbidity in hypertension: results in patients with diastolic blood pressures averaging 115 through 129 mmHg. *JAMA* 1967; **202**:1028–1034.

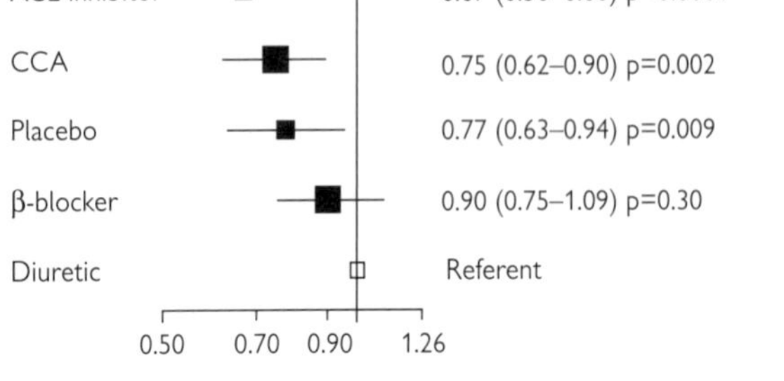

Fig. 7.5 Relative risk of developing new-onset diabetes for different classes of antihypertensive drug. Reprinted from Elliott WJ and Meyer PM (2007). Incident diabetes in clinical trials of antihypertensive drugs: a network meta-analysis. *Lancet* **369**:201–7, © 2007 with permission from Elsevier.

Potassium-sparing diuretics

Agents

Only 2 agents are available in the UK: amiloride and triamterene (rarely used). They are relatively weak diuretics, and may be used alone or in combination with other diuretics to maintain plasma K^+. Usual dose of amiloride 2.5–10mg OD, although higher doses may be used in hyperaldosteronism.

Mechanism of action

Inhibit Na^+ uptake in the distal tubule (📖 Fig. 7.6) by blocking the ENaC. This results in less Na^+ reabsorption, and consequently less K^+ excretion (passively via the ROMK channel). The hypotensive effect is thought to be due to a combination of reduced extra-cellular volume and a direct vasodilator action.

Evidence base

There are no large RCT of K^+-sparing diuretics, but a number of smaller trials suggest roughly equivalent BP ↓ to other antihypertensive agents.

Indications

They may be used to maintain plasma K^+ levels, or in the treatment of hyperaldosteronism, when considerably larger doses may be required. They may also be effective in synergy with other diuretics or ACEIs/ARAs (care with K^+ levels) in the management of low-renin patients.

Compelling indications

- Hyperaldosteronism.

Contra-indications

- Hyperkalaemia.
- Renal failure.

Side effects

- Hyperkalaemia.
- GI upset.
- Dry mouth.
- Postural hypotension.

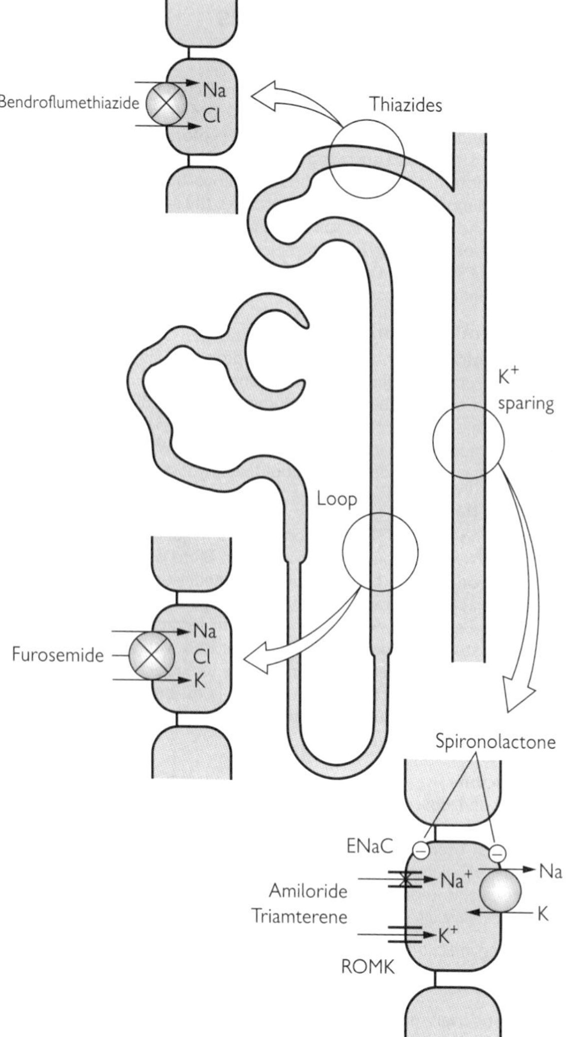

Fig. 7.6 Site of action of the diuretics used to treat hypertension.

Aldosterone antagonists

Agents

Two agents are licensed in the UK: spironolactone and the newer drug eplerenone. Spironolactone is less specific than eplerenone, partly blocking androgen and activating progesterone receptors—which accounts for some of its side effects such as gynaecomastia. However, spironolactone is a more potent antagonist at the mineralocorticoid receptor, and high doses of eplerenone are required to produce the same degree of receptor blockade. The usual dose of spironolactone is 25–100mg OD. Low doses (25–50mg) seem as effective as higher doses (>100mg) for most patients, and produce fewer side effects, although considerably higher doses may be needed in hyperaldosteronism.

Mechanism of action

Block the intra-cellular aldosterone receptor, thus antagonizing the salt- and water-retaining effects of aldosterone (📖 Fig. 7.7). This leads to a reduction in extra-cellular fluid volume and fall in BP. It has also been suggested that aldosterone blockade may prevent or reverse cardiac and vascular remodelling, particularly fibrosis which may be important in end-organ damage and the development of fixed hypertension.

Evidence base

There are no large RCTs of aldosterone antagonists, but a number of smaller trials suggest roughly equivalent ↓ in BP to other antihypertensive agents. Spironolactone has been used in combination with thiazides diuretics or as add-on therapy in a number of large studies including ASCOT and appears effective, even in subjects with refractory hypertension. In the RALES study, spironolactone was associated with a significant reduction in events when given as add-on therapy to subjects with heart failure. Eplerenone seems effective in reducing BP in essential hypertension, and also reduces events in subjects with heart failure post-MI (EPHESUS).

Indications

Spironolactone is routinely used in the management of hyperaldosteronism, and doses of up to 200mg may be required. It is undergoing something of a renaissance in the management of essential hypertension, and is often used as add-on therapy in resistant cases. It is particularly effective in subjects with low-renin hypertension, such as older people and blacks, and in diabetics. It has also been advocated for subjects with polycystic ovary disease and those with the metabolic syndrome.

Compelling indications

- Hyperaldosteronism.
- Blacks.
- Polycystic ovary disease

Contra-indications

- Hyperkalaemia.
- Hyponatraemia.
- Renal failure.

Side effects

- Hyperkalaemia—more common if chronic renal failure or diabetic.
- GI upset.
- Impotence.
- Gynaecomastia.

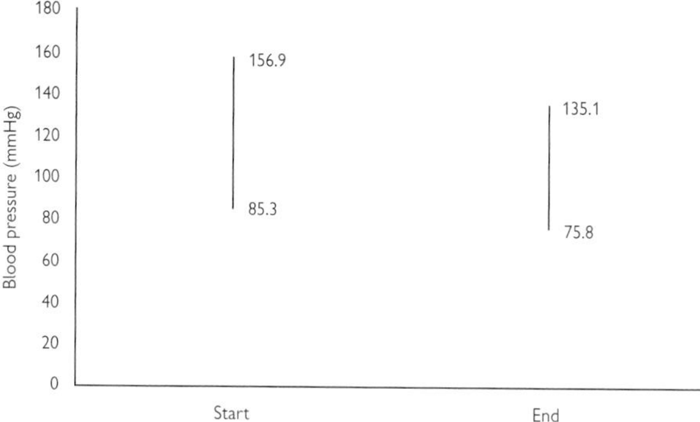

Fig. 7.7 Effect of spironolactone on resistant hypertensive subjects in the ASCOT Study (average dose 25mg). Data from Chapman N, *et al.* (2007). Effect of spironolactone on blood pressure in subjects with resistant hypertension *Hypertension* **49**:839–45.

Alpha-blockers

Agents

Non-selective α-blockers include phentolamine and phenoxybenzamine. Phentolamine is mainly used in the management of hypertensive crisis associated with catecholamine excess. Phenoxybenzamine, a non-competitive, irreversible, antagonist, is used in the chronic management of phaeochromocytoma. α_1-selective antagonists include prazosin, indoramin, terazosin, and doxazosin. Prazosin is now seldom used due to a relatively short $t_{1/2}$, which can lead to rapid reductions in BP. Most BP reduction occurs at low-mid dose: usual dose of doxazosin is 1–8mg OD, titrated slowly, or 4–8mg of the slow-release preparation.

Mechanism of action

Antagonists at α-adrenoceptors: α_1-adrenoceptors are predominantly post-synaptic and mediate catecholamine-induced vasoconstriction. α_2-adrenoceptors are mainly pre-synaptic and inhibit neuronal catecholamine release. BP ↓ results from peripheral vasodilatation, and there tends to be concomitant salt and water retention with high doses (↑ renin). Non-selective α-blockers tend to ↑ central sympathetic drive (via α_2 inhibition) which results in a reflex tachycardia and more marked elevation in renin. Thus, α_1-selective are usually used in essential hypertension.

Evidence base

As effective in reducing BP as most of the other main classes of antihypertensive drug; seem slightly more effective in low-mid renin states. The doxazosin-arm of the ALLHAT study was stopped prematurely due to an excess of heart failure (66%) and CVD (25%) compared with those randomized to chlortalidone (📖 Fig. 7.8). However, there was no difference in the 1° endpoint of MI or overall mortality. Nevertheless, this led most groups to suggest that α_1-blockers were used as add-on therapy rather than 1st-line.

Indications

Rarely used as monotherapy now, but can be combined with all the major classes of antihypertensive. May be particularly useful in subjects with prostatism—help to reduce outflow obstruction. α_1-blockers have a mild insulin-sensitizing effect, and may slightly improve the lipid profile.

Compelling indications

- Prostatism.

Contra-indications

- Caution in patients with heart failure.

Side effects

- ► Care with 1st dose: may case profound hypotension.
- Postural hypotension.
- Drowsiness.
- Headache.
- Rhinitis.

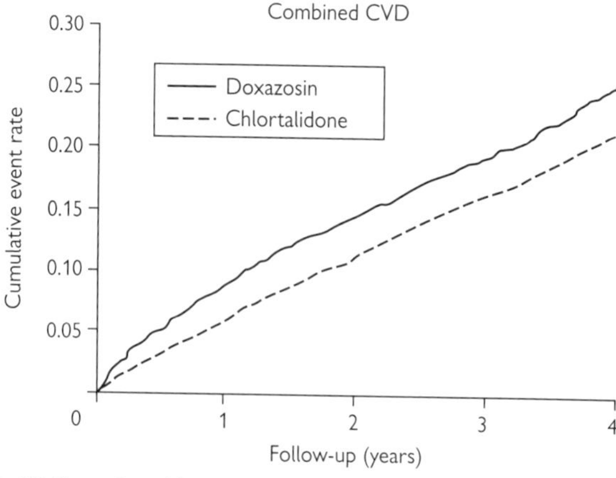

Fig. 7.8 Comparison of doxazosin and chlortalidone in the ALLHAT study. There was a significant excess of CV events (and heart failure) in those receiving doxazosin. Reproduced with permission from The ALLHAT Officers and Coordinators for the ALLHAT Collaborative Research Group (2000). Major cardiovascular events in hypertensive patients randomized to doxazosin vs. chlortalidone: The Antihypertensive and Lipid-Lowering Treatment to Prevent Heart Attack Trial (ALLHAT). *JAMA* **283**:1967–75.

Renin inhibitors

Agents

Direct renin-inhibitors are the newest class of antihypertensives. Aliskiren is the only available agent in the UK and was licensed in 2007, following many years of research for an orally active agent. Usual dose is 150–300mg OD.

Mechanism of action

Renin is an enzyme that cleaves circulating angiotensinogen to angiotensin I (📖 Fig. 7.9). Direct renin inhibitors bind to renin and reduce its enzymatic activity. This leads to lower levels of circulating angiotensin II and aldosterone, and consequently vasodilatation and a reduction in extra-cellular volume.

Evidence base

Head-to-head comparisons demonstrate that aliskiren produces equivalent BP ↓ to the main other antihypertensive drugs. It is also produces additional BP ↓ when used in combination—even with an ACEI or ARA. As yet there are no comparative outcome studies with aliskiren.

Indications

Likely to be useful in patients with an activated renin–angiotensin system, and may be of benefit in reducing proteinuria (studies awaited).

Contra-indications

- Pregnancy.

Side effects

- Hyperkalaemia.
- Diarrhoea.

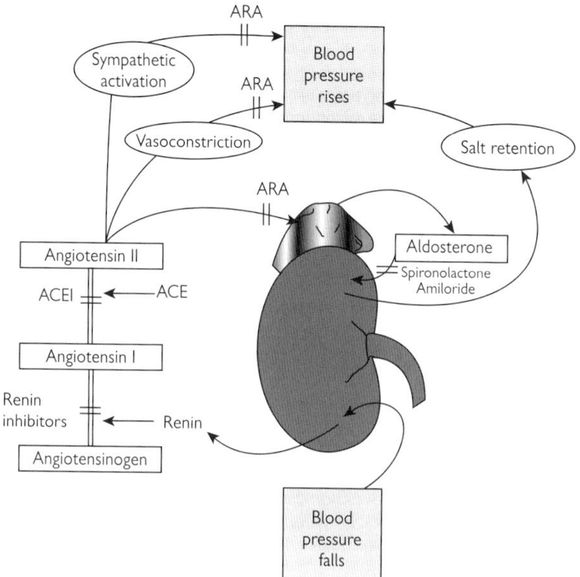

Fig. 7.9 The renin–angiotensin system.

Central sympatholytics

Agents

Centrally-acting sympatholytics were amongst the 1st drugs used to treat hypertension, but, with the exception of moxonidine, are now rarely used due to an adverse side-effect profile. 3 drugs fall into this class: methyldopa, moxonidine, and clonidine. Methyldopa is still widely used in pregnancy due to a proven safety profile; usual dose 250mg to 1g TDS. Moxonidine is less sedating; usual dose 200–400mcg OD. Clonidine can be administered IV or PO but must be withdrawn slowly to avoid hypertensive crisis; usual dose 50–200mcgTDS PO.

Mechanism of action

All 3 drugs reduce central sympathetic outflow, thereby lowering PVR. Cardiac output tends to remain the same or ↓ slightly. Methyldopa is taken up by sympathetic neurons and converted into α-methylnoradrenaline, which is then concentrated into vesicles and released. α-methylnoradrenaline is a false transmitter: being inactive at α_1-adrenoceptors, but is an agonist at presynaptic α_2-adrenoceptors, thus inhibiting its own release. Moxonidine is a selective I_1-imidazoline receptor agonist and is thought to act mainly in the rostral ventrolateral medulla oblongata to reduce sympathetic outflow. Clonidine is an α_2-adrenoceptor agonist with some action at I_1-receptors. However, at high doses it becomes an agonist at the α_1-adrenoceptor, paradoxically ↑ BP.

Evidence base

Centrally-acting sympatholytics have been included in a number of antihypertensive studies mainly as add-on therapy but have not been the focus of large RCT.

Indications

Methyldopa is safe in pregnancy and frequently used despite its adverse side-effect profile. Clonidine is rarely used except IV in ITU or theatre. Moxonidine may be used as add-on therapy in resistant patients. Theoretically, centrally-acting drugs may be useful in patients with sympathetic activation including those with the 'metabolic syndrome'.

Contra-indications

- Depression, acute liver disease, phaeochromocytoma (methyldopa).
- Conduction defects, severe heart failure, angio-oedema (moxonidine).

Side effects

- Dry mouth.
- Postural hypotension.
- Depression.
- Haemolytic anaemia (methyldopa).
- Liver dysfunction (methyldopa).

►Always withdraw clonidine slowly to avoid a hypertensive crisis.

Sodium nitroprusside

SNP is a nitrovasodilator drug, which spontaneously decomposes *in vivo* to release NO. Only used for the management of hypertensive emergencies such as encephalopathy. Given by continuous IV infusion, and capable of producing rapid and profound reductions in BP. Intra-arterial BP monitoring is essential. The compound and solution must be protected from light as this ↑ the rate of decomposition.

Side effects

- Tachycardia.
- Headache.
- Excessive ↓ BP.

►Cyanide toxicity may occur, especially with prolonged infusion due to a build-up of the cyanide metabolite. This may lead to tachycardia, sweating, hyperventilation etc.: stop the infusion and administer cyanide antidote.

Minoxidil

A potent direct vasodilator (opens adenosine triphosphate-sensitive potassium channels in vascular smooth muscle cells). BP ↓ is due to a substantial reduction in peripheral resistance. However, this leads to a reflex tachycardia and activation of the renin–angiotensin system with resultant salt and water retention, which tends to offset the BP fall leading to pseudotolerance. For this reason, and to reduce side effects (ankle oedema and palpitations), all but the smallest doses of minoxidil require concomitant use of β-blockers and loop diuretics (often 80–120mg of furosemide a day).

Largely reserved for the management of resistant hypertension due to its side-effect profile. It is unusual to find a patient unresponsive to the introduction of minoxidil if adequately β-blocked and salt and water retention are prevented. Usual dose: 5–40mg per day.

Contra-indications

- Phaeochromocytoma.

Side effects

- Peripheral oedema, weight gain.
- Tachycardia.
- Excessive hair growth.
- LVH and myocardial ischaemia (especially if not combined with a β-blocker).

Hydralazine

A less potent direct vasodilator than minoxidil, with an unknown mechanism of action. Introduced for the management of hypertension in the 1950s but now rarely used outside obstetrics due to pseudotolerance and an adverse side-effect profile. Occasionally still used in resistant hypertension.

When used orally for resistant hypertension it is often combined with a β-blocker and loop diuretic. Usual dose: 25–50mg QDS (start with 25mg BD). Higher doses dramatically increase the risk of side effects.

IV infusion may be used in a hypertensive crisis –especially pre-eclampsia. Usual dose range 50–150mcg/min.

Contra-indications

- Systemic lupus erythematosus
- Severe tachycardia.

Side effects

- Tachycardia, fluid retention.
- Flushing, headache.
- Rashes, peripheral neuritis.
- Lupus-like syndrome—especially women and slow acetylators.

► Metabolism is genetically determined, and fast acetylators have fewer side effects.

Nitrates

Organic nitrate such as isosorbide dinitrate are unlicensed for the treatment of essential hypertension and have not been subject to outcome trials in hypertensives. However, they do lower BP and may be particularly useful in older subjects with ISH as they act mainly on SBP at low doses, due to venodilatation and a reduction in wave reflection. DBP tends to be little affected. Moreover, the effect on aortic systolic pressure is even more pronounced than that observed at the brachial artery. Similarly they may be double benefit in subjects with angina.

Although, theoretically, tolerance is an issue with continued oral administration, this is not supported by the few RCTs that have been conducted (📖 Fig. 7.10). The usual dose is 20–40mg BD of isosorbide dinitrate MR.

Side effects

- Headache.
- Flushing.
- Postural hypotension.

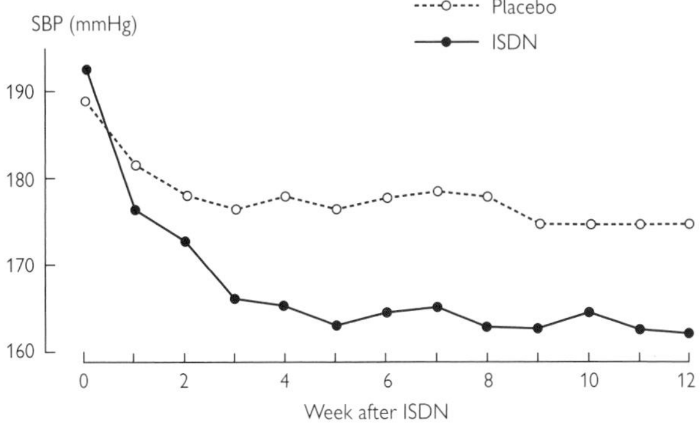

Fig. 7.10 Isosorbide dinitrate (ISDN) produces a sustained reduction in systolic pressure in subjects with ISH. Redrawn from Duchier J, Safar M (1987) Autocrine-paracrine mechanisms of vascular myocytes in systematic hypertension. *Am J Cardiol* **60**:99–102, with permission from Elsevier.

Other agents

Peripheral sympatholytics

Guanethidine and reserpine (now withdrawn in the UK) block noradrenaline release from postganglionic sympathetic neurons by depleting vesicles of catecholamines. Although effective in reducing BP they are now rarely used due to their side-effect profile. In particular, they impair the ability to respond to postural haemodynamic changes, and may lead to postural hypotension. Other side effects include nasal stuffiness, failure of ejaculation, and drowsiness. Reserpine also has a CNS action and may lead to depression. They should not be used in conjunction with MAOIs as they may precipitate a hypertensive crisis.

Endothelin antagonists

Endothelin-1 is a potent long-lasting vasopressor, and a range of ET_A selective or mixed ET_A/ET_B receptor antagonists have been synthesized and trialled in human essential hypertension. Although moderately effective in reducing BP, they have not been developed further due to concerns over side effects and teratogenicity. However, a number are available for use in pulmonary hypertension

Chapter 8

Hypertension in the 21st century

Prevention

Hypertension is a major cause of morbidity and mortality throughout the world. This carries considerable economic cost, and treatment is set to rise as the developing nations adapt and adopt modern lifestyles and more people receive treatment.

One of the main ways in reducing this burden would be prevention. We have examined the effects of diet and exercise, weight loss, ↓ Na^+ and ↑ K^+ intake, stress reduction, as well as pharmacological methods on BP in 📖 Chapter 2, but the issue of hypertension prevention using these methods has not been addressed yet in clinical trials—mainly as it has not shown long-lasting effects, either due to a failure to comply or a lack of sustained effort in maintenance of these non-pharmacological methods.

Only 1 trial has examined the effects of prevention of onset hypertension using pharmacological means; this was the Trial of Prevention Hypertension (TROPHY). 800 pre-hypertensive adults (mean age 49, SBP 130–139mmHg, DBP ≤89mmHg or SBP ≤139mmHg and DBP 85–89mmHg) were randomized in a double-blind manner to 2 years of candesartan 16mg OD or placebo and then all patients were put on placebo for a further 2 years.

New hypertension developed in 40% of placebo but only 13% of the candesartan group in the first 2 years (66% RR reduction in favour of candesartan group), but at 4 years the percentages were 63% and 53% (a 16 % RR reduction for the candesartan group).

Critics argue that the pre-treatment in the active arm masked the onset of hypertension and that the incidence of hypertension in the final 2 years was not different between the groups. Moreover, given that BP is a continuous variable, it is perhaps not surprising that an antihypertensive drug ↓ BP in prehypertensives whilst they remain on it. New, more aggressive strategies ought to be explored in perhaps younger subjects.

Cardiovascular risk assessment

There are a number of tools to help determine CV risk (📖 see Prognosis and risk stratification, pp.84–87). These are useful to predict a 10-year risk based on variables such as age, gender, cholesterol, and BP.

A lot of the data are based on Framingham datasets and these are not applicable to various cohorts of people. The data were based on Caucasian populations—therefore they cannot really translate across to other races. In addition, they require pre-treatment baseline values, which are not always obtainable. Current risk therefore is indeterminable using these methods. They do not predict risk in children, the young, in pregnancy, or situations of accelerated hypertensive states.

Most importantly, there is a bias towards treatment of the elderly in these methods, thereby minimizing the lifetime risk associated with a CV event 20 or 30 years in the future. This may occur in the younger patient with a constellation of minimally raised risk factors, all of which are borderline and not requiring therapy. This negates the importance of non-pharmacological interventions, such as a healthy diet and exercise, until atherosclerosis has probably already begun.

Therefore, efforts need to be focused on developing new tools which assess risk continually and on current therapy. This may be a composite of biomarkers and physiological parameters which give an individual risk score, rather than one centred on population-based datasets. In addition, an individual's lifetime risk should be the focus of initiating management of risk early on, rather than waiting for the atherosclerotic process to set in.

Dilemmas in modern management

There are a few areas which, despite the trials that have been conducted, have not been fully understood or evaluated.

Target blood pressure

Over the last 3 decades, the target BP has gradually reduced as ↑ evidence points to a ↓ BP as being a major determinant of length of life. This is largely based on 1 study, namely HOT—which was essentially negative for its 1° outcome and failed to achieve target BPs of the study. Although BP is continuously related to risk down to 115/70mmHg, we need evidence if lower pressures are better; this may be addressed in the SPRINT trial. A concept that has not yet emerged—but is likely to—is that of an age-related target BP. This would require a lot more research, adjusting for a variety of factors including race, salt intake, gender, and so on.

Borderline hypertension

The diagnosis of hypertension is arbitrary and there is a continuum of risk, but where the boundary lies between normality and a diagnosis of hypertension continues to mean that a cohort of people remain at risk but have to achieve TOD before therapy is instituted. This may have important consequences in the longer term, and therefore is an important area in younger people with borderline hypertension. The usual rules for initiating therapy in this cohort of patients mean that their lifetime risk of an event is underestimated by the lack of fluidity within current guidelines.

2° hypertension

There is still a huge debate on whether every patient diagnosed with hypertension should undergo a battery of tests to rule out 2° causes. One the one hand, this would be advantageous, since the earlier a cause is found, the more likely a cure is likely to benefit the patient. However, as it is such a common condition, and 80–90% is still defined as essential hypertension, critics argue this is not a cost-effective investigation. More economical tests and guidelines which stratify which cohorts of patients require further evaluation are currently being introduced to help this process.

BP measurement site

The debate as to whether brachial BP, which has long been the standard measurement of BP, should, in fact be replaced by newer methods of predicting and measuring central aortic BP, continues as the evidence for the latter grows. The fact that wave reflections and the stiffness of the vascular tree contribute to varying central BP, independent of brachial BP, means that this will continue to be the focus of this century's research in hypertension.

Emerging concepts: arterial stiffness

The large elastic arteries act to cushion the highly pulsatile blood flow resulting from intermittent cardiac ejection, by expanding during systole and providing elastic recoil during diastole. However, in almost all societies worldwide, there is progressive stiffening of the large arteries with age, resulting in a widening of the pulse pressure and leading to the development of ISH, as well as a number of other adverse haemodynamic consequences (📖 see Isolated systolic hypertension, p.52). CV risk factors such as hypertension, hypercholesterolaemia, smoking, and diabetes are also associated with ↑ arterial stiffness, leading to the notion that individuals with such risk factors experience premature vascular ageing. Moreover, aortic stiffness is now recognized as an important, independent, determinant of CV risk in a variety of patient groups (📖 Table 8.1).

Arterial stiffness can be assessed using a variety of different techniques. These broadly fall into measures of stiffness at one discrete location, e.g. ultrasound-derived distensibility and compliance; or more regional measures, such as the pulse wave velocity. This is a measure of the speed with which the pressure waveform propagates along a segment of the arterial tree; the stiffer the vessel the faster the wave travels. The aortic pulse wave velocity is often considered as the current 'gold-standard' measure of arterial stiffness.

An ↑ in arterial stiffness also ↑ the speed at which pressure waves are reflected back towards the heart from major bifurcations and sites of vascular impedance mismatch. When such reflected waves arrive back in the ascending aorta in early systole, they augment the central (aortic) systolic pressure (augmentation pressure). The contribution of reflected pressure waves to central pressure is quantified by the augmentation index, which is itself, an independent determinant of CV risk. There is a progressive ↑ in augmentation pressure and, therefore, central pressure, with ageing. This explains why the difference between peripheral and central pressure is more marked in younger individuals than in older individuals, as discussed in Chapter 1 (📖 see Central versus peripheral blood pressure, p.6).

Clinical use

Pulse wave velocity, augmentation index, and central pressure are all independent determinants of CV risk. However, the wide-spread adoption of these measurements into routine clinical practice will ultimately depend on the availability of appropriate devices and the development of guidelines on which clinical decisions may be based. The most recent ESH/ESC guidelines for the management of hypertension recommend measuring the aortic pulse wave velocity. A value of 12m/s has been identified as a threshold with which to identify the presence of sub-clinical organ damage. Further research is required to identify appropriate treatment thresholds for pulse wave velocity, augmentation index, and central BP.

Table 8.1 Longitudinal studies reporting the independent predictive value of arterial stiffness, according to the site of measurement*

Measurement site	First author (year, country)	Events	Follow-up (years)	Type of patient (number)
Aortic PWV	Blacher (1999, Fr)	CV mortality	6.0	ESRD (241)
	Laurent (2001, Fr)	CV mortality	9.3	Hypertension (1980)
	Meaume (2001, Fr)	CV mortality	2.5	Elderly (>70) (141)
	Shoji (2001, Jp)	CV mortality	5.2	ESRD (265)
	Boutouyrie (2002, Fr)	CHD events	5.7	Hypertension (1045)
	Cruickshank (2002, GB)	All cause mortality	10.7	IGT (571)
	Laurent (2003, Fr)	Fatal strokes	7.9	Hypertension (1715)
	Sutton-Tyrrell (2005, USA)	CV mortality and events	4.6	Elderly (2488)
	Shokawa (2005, Jp)	CV mortality	10	General population (492)
	Willum-Hansen (2006, Dk)	CV mortality	9.4	General population (1678)
	Mattace-Raso (2006, Neth.)	CV mt, CHD	4.1	Elderly (2835)
Ascending aorta (invasive)	Stefanadis (2000, Gr)	Recurrent acute CHD	3	Acute CHD (54)
Carotid distensibility	Blacher (1998, Fr)	All cause mortality	2.1	ESRD (79)
	Barenbrock (2001, Ge)	CV events	7.9	ESRD (68)

ESRD, end-stage renal disease; Fr, France; GB, Great Britain; Ge, Germany; Gr, Greece; Neth, The Netherlands; PWV, pulse wave velocity; USA, United States of America.

*Reproduced with permission from Laurent S, *et al.* (2006) Expert consensus document on arterial stiffness: methodological issues and clinical applications. *Eur Heart J* **27**:2588–605.

Table 8.2 Recommended clinical variables to stratify total CV risk*

Risk factors	Subclinical organ damage

• Systolic and diastolic BP levels
• Levels of pulse pressure (in the elderly)
• Age (M > 55 years; W > 65 years)
• Smoking
• Dyslipidaemia
  • TC > 5.0 mmol/l (190 mg/dl)
  or:
  • LDL-C > 3.0 mmol/l (115mg/dl)
  or:
  • HDL-C: M < 1.0 mmol/l (40 mg/dl)
  • W < 1.2 mmol/; (46 mg/dl)
  or:
  • TG > 1.7 mmol/l (150 mg/dl)
• Fasting plasma glucose 5.6–6.9 mmol/l (102–125 mg/dl)
• Abnormal glucose tolerance test
• Abdominal obesity (waist circumference > 102 cm (M), > 88 cm (W))
• Family history of premature CV disease (M at age < 55 years; W at age < 65 years)
	• Electrocardiographic LVH (Sokolow-Lyon > 38 mm; Cornell > 2440 mm/ms)
	or:
	• Echocardiographic LVH ♦ (LVMIM ≥ 125 g/m2, W ≥ 110 g/m²)
	• Carotid wall thickening (IMT > 0.9 mm) or plaque
	• Carotid-femoral pulse wave velocity > 12 m/sec
	• Ankle/Brachial BP index < 0.9
	• Slight increase in plasma creatinine: M: 115–133 µmol/l (1.3–1.5 mg/dl) W: 107–124 µmol/l (1.2–1.4 mg/dl)
	• Low estimated glomerular filtration rate ♦♦ (< 60 ml/min.1.73 m²) or creatinine clearance ♦♦♦ (< 60 ml/min)
	• Microalbuminuria 30–300 mg/24 h or albumin-creatinine ratio: ≥ 22 (M); or ≥ 31 (W) mg/g creatinine

Diabetes mellitus	**Established CV or renal disease**
• Fasting plasma glucose ≥ 7.0 mmol/l (126 mg/dl) on repeated measurement or: • Postload plasma glucose > 11.0 mmol/l (198 mg/dl) Note: the cluster of three out of 5 risk factors among abdominal, obesity, altered tasting plasma glucose, BP ≥ 130/85 mmHg, low HDL cholesterol and high TG (as defined above) indicates the presence of metabolic syndrome.	• Cerebrovascular disease: ischaemic stroke; cerebral haemorrhage; transient ischaemic attack • Heart disease: myocardial infarction; angina; coronary revascularization; heart failure • Renal disease: diabetic nephropathy; renal impairment (serum creatinine M > 133; W > 124 µmol/l); proteinuria (> 300 mg/24 h) • Peripheral artery disease • Advanced retinopathy: haemorrhages or exudates, papilloedema

*Reproduced with permission from Mancia G, *et al.* (2007). 2007 ESH-ESC Practice Guidelines for the Management of Arterial Hypertension: ESH-ESC Task Force on the Management of Arterial Hypertension. *J Hypertens* **25**:1751–62.

Useful websites

- American College of Cardiology: 🖱 http://www.acc.org/
- American Heart Association: 🖱 http://www.americanheart.org/
- American Society of Hypertension: 🖱 http://www.ash-us.org/
- British Cardiovascular Society: 🖱 http://www.bcs.com/pages/default.asp
- British Heart Foundation: 🖱 http://www.bhf.org.uk/
- British Hypertension Society: 🖱 http://www.bhsoc.org/
- European Society of Hypertension: 🖱 http://www.eshonline.org/
- European Society of Cardiology: 🖱 http://www.escardio.org/Pages/index.aspx
- International Society of Hypertension: 🖱 http://www.ish-world.com
- Phaeochromocytoma Research Organisation: 🖱 http://www.pressor.org/

Clinical trials: a glossary

The rest of this chapter provides a summary of all the major clinical trials listed (as acronyms or otherwise) in this book and some other landmark trials related to hypertension and CVD.

Whilst this is not an extensive list, we hope it provides some useful points about each trial and highlights the important milestones achieved as a result of these trials.

ABCD

Trial name

Appropriate Blood Pressure Control in Diabetes.

Reference

NEJM 1998; **338**:645–52.

Design

Prospective, randomized, double blind.

Sample size (n)

950.

Question addressed

Effect of moderate vs. intensive BP control using either enalapril (ACEI) or nisoldipine (CCA) in NIDDM patients (normotensive and hypertensive) on complications of diabetes.

1°endpoint

Morbidity.

Results

2° endpoint of CV outcome showed a significant reduction in MI rates with those on enalapril than on nisoldipine in the hypertensive cohort (both in the moderate and intensive arms of BP reduction).

ACE

Trial name

Aspirin and Carotid Endarterectomy.

Reference

Lancet 1999; **353**:2179–84.

Design

Randomized, double-blind, parallel-group.

Sample size (n)

2849.

Question addressed

Effect of high- vs. low-dose aspirin (ASA) on stroke rates in carotid endarterectomy.

1°endpoint

Mortality and morbidity.

Results

Low-dose ASA (81 or 325mg) had a lower incidence of stroke, MI, and death than high-dose at 30 days (5.4% vs. 7.0%; $p = 0.07$) and at 3 months (6.2% vs. 8.4%; $p = 0.03$). A posthoc analysis showed greater differences when patients taking high-dose ASA before randomization and patients randomized within 1 day of surgery: combined incidences in the low-dose and high-dose groups were 3.7% and 8.2% at 30 days ($p = 0.002$) and 4.2% and 10.0% at 3 months ($p = 0.0002$).

AIRE

Trial name

Acute Infarction Ramipril Efficacy study.

Reference

Lancet 1993; **342**:821–8.

Design

RCT, double-blind, placebo-controlled, parallel-group.

Sample size (n)

2006.

Questions addressed

- 1°: effect of ramipril on total mortality in patients surviving acute MI with early clinical evidence of heart failure.
- 2°: effect of ramipril on progression of heart failure, non-fatal reinfarction and stroke between the 2 groups.

1°endpoint

Mortality.

Results

Ramipril reduced total mortality by 27% ($p = 0.002$), sudden death by 30% ($p = 0.011$) and death from circulatory failure by 18% ($p = 0.237$). There was no change to stroke or non-fatal reinfarction.

ALLHAT

Trial name

Antihypertensive and Lipid-Lowering treatment to prevent Heart Attack Trial.

Reference

JAMA 2002; **288**:2891–97 and 2998–3007.

Design

- Antihypertensive arm: randomized, double-blind.
- Lipid-lowering arm (LLA): randomized, open.

Sample size (n)

- Antihypertensive arm: 33,357 aged ≥55 years with hypertension and at least 1 other risk factor for CHD.
- LLA: 10,355 aged ≥55 years, fasting LDL cholesterol 3.1–4.9mmol/L (patients without CHD) or 2.6–3.3mmol/L (with known CHD), and fasting TG levels <3.9mmol/L.

Questions addressed

- Antihypertensive arm: incidence of fatal and non-fatal MI in patients treated with chlortalidone, amlodipine, lisinopril, or doxazosin.
- LLA: all-cause mortality in patients treated with either pravastatin or 'usual care'

1° endpoint

Mortality and morbidity.

Results

- Antihypertensive arm: No significant difference was observed between drugs. Events occurred in 2956 patients.
  - Amlodipine (RR 0.98, 95% CI 0.90–1.07; p = 0.65) or lisinopril (RR 0.99, 95% CI 0.91–1.08; p = 0.81) vs. chlortalidone.
  - Doxazosin arm discontinued prematurely for possible ↑ incidence of heart failure.
- LLA: all-cause mortality did not differ significantly between the pravastatin and usual care treatment groups (RR 0.99, 95% CI 0.89–1.11; p = 0.88).

ALPINE

Trial name
Antihypertensive Treatment and Lipid Profile in a North of Sweden Efficacy Evaluation.

Reference
J Hypertens 2003; **21**:1563–74.

Design
Randomized, double-blind, controlled, parallel-group.

Sample size (n)
392.

Questions addressed
Metabolic outcomes of treatment with low-dose diuretic (hydrochlorothiazide, HCTZ), alone (or in combination with atenolol), with that of an angiotensin II type 1 receptor blocker (candesartan), alone (or in combination with felodipine), in newly diagnosed patients with 1° hypertension.

1° endpoint
Morbidity.

Results
Despite similar BP reductions, fasting serum insulin and plasma glucose levels ↑ in the HCTZ group unlike the candesartan group. Diabetes mellitus was diagnosed in 4.1% of the HCTZ group and 0.5% in the candesartan group ($p = 0.03$). The LDL:HDL was worse in the HCTZ group and conversely in the candesartan group ($p < 0.01$). TG was ↑ in HCTZ group ($p < 0.001$).

ANBP2

Trial name
Australian National Blood Pressure study 2.

Reference
NEJM 2003; **348**:583–92.

Design
Randomized, open.

Sample size (n)
6083.

Questions addressed
Difference in total CV events (fatal and non-fatal) between ACEI vs. diuretic-based regimen over a 5-year treatment period in 65–84-year-old hypertensives.

1° endpoint
Mortality.

Results
There were fewer deaths in the ACEI-based arm than diuretic group ($p = 0.05$) and non-fatal CV events ($p = 0.03$). This was evident more so in men.

ASCOT

Trial name

Anglo-Scandinavian Cardiac Outcomes Trial

References

Lancet 2003; **361**:1149–58.
Lancet 2005; **366**:895–906.

Design

- Antihypertensive arm: randomized, parallel-group, 2 × 2 factorial.
- LLA: double-blind, placebo-controlled, 2 × 2 factorial.

Sample size (n)

- Antihypertensive arm: 19,257 mean age 63 years, with BP ≥160/100mmHg untreated or ≥140/90mmHg treated + ≥3 of 11 specified CV risk factors.
- LLA: 10,305 with total cholesterol ≤6.5mmol/L and a TC:HDL cholesterol ratio ≤4.5.

Questions addressed

- Antihypertensive arm: non-fatal MI and fatal CHD rates of a old regimen (atenolol ± bendroflumethiazide) vs. new regimen (amlodipine ± perindopril) in hypertensive patients,
- LLA: atorvastatin vs. placebo in hypertensive patients with dyslipidaemia.

1° endpoint

Mortality and morbidity.

Results

- Antihypertensive arm: no significant difference between the groups: 4.5% of patients in the amlodipine group compared to 4.9% of patients in the atenolol group (hazard ratio (HR) 0.90, 95% CI 0.79−1.02; p = 0.1052). However, fatal and non-fatal stroke, total CV events/ procedures, and all-cause mortality were significantly better in the amlodipine group, as was the incidence of diabetes.
- LLA: significant difference in 1° endpoint: 1.9% of patients in the atorv-astatin group compared to 3.0% in the placebo group (HR 0.64, 95% CI 0.50−0.83; p = 0.0005).

ASTRAL

Trial name

Angioplasty and Stent for Renal Artery Lesions.

Reference

J Hum Hypertens 2007; **21**:511–15 (study design). Formal results yet to be published.

Design

Randomized.

Sample size (n)

806.

Question addressed

Does renal artery stenting for atherosclerotic renovascular disease offer more benefits than medical therapy?

1° endpoint

Decline in renal function over time.

Results (preliminary)

No difference in the levels of renal function between those allocated a stent vs. medical management. There were also no differences in the 2° endpoints of blood pressure, first MI, stroke, vascular death, hospitalization for angina, fluid overload, and cardiac failure. 3% of the stent patients had experienced a procedure-related complication.

CAFE

Trial name

Conduit Artery Function Evaluation.

Reference

Circulation 2006; **113**;1213–25.

Design

Randomized, parallel group.

Sample size (n)

2073.

Questions addressed

- 1°: ASCOT substudy testing the hypothesis that the effects of antihypertensives differ in their effects on central pressures despite similar brachial pressures.
- 2°: these differences in central pressure explains differences in CV outcomes.

1° endpoint

Physiological endpoint.

Results

Antihypertensives have differing effects on central BP despite similar brachial BP. Central aortic pulse pressure and differences in central pressure may explain differences in CV outcomes despite similar brachial BP changes.

CAPPP

Trial name
Captopril Prevention Project.

Reference
Lancet 1999; **353**:611–16.

Design
Prospective randomized open blinded endpoint (PROBE).

Sample size (n)
10,985.

Question addressed
Does captopril treatment differ in CV outcomes compared to conventional antihypertensives (diuretics and β-blockers)?

1° endpoint
Mortality and morbidity.

Results
The 1° endpoint for fatal/non-fatal MI and stroke, and other CV deaths was negative. The study had 698 events in total.

CHARM

Trial name

Candesartan in Heart failure: Assessment of Reduction in Mortality and morbidity – Overall.

Reference

Lancet 2003; **362**:759–66.

Design

Randomized, double-blind, placebo-controlled, parallel-group.

Sample size (n)

7599.

Question addressed

Effects of an angiotensin-receptor blocker on mortality and morbidity in chronic heart failure.

1° endpoint

Mortality and morbidity.

Results

CV deaths were fewer in the candesartan group than in the placebo group (HR 0.88, 95% CI 0.79–0.97; p = 0.012). Time to CV death or hospital admission for worsening chronic heart failure was reduced by 16% (30% with candesartan and 35% with placebo; p <0.0001). No change in total mortality from any cause.

DASH

Trial name
Dietary Approaches to Stop Hypertension.

Reference
NEJM 1997; **336**:1117–24.

Design
Randomized, controlled.

Sample size (n)
459.

Question addressed
To assess the effects of dietary patterns on BP.

1° endpoint
BP.

Results
- Compared to the control diet, the combination diet significantly reduced BP 5.5/3mmHg (both p <0.001), while the fruit and vegetable diet reduced BP by 2.8/1.1mmHg.
- Compared to the fruit and vegetable diet, the combination diet reduced BP by 2.7/1.9mmHg.
- In the hypertensive group, the combination diet reduced BP by 11.4/5.5mmHg compared to the control diet (both p <0.001).
- The corresponding additional reductions were 3.5mmHg (p <0.001) and 2.1mmHg (p = 0.003), respectively, in the normotensive subjects.

DRASTIC

Trial name

Dutch Renal Artery Stenosis Intervention Cooperative study.

References

NEJM 2000; **342**:1007–14.
J Hum Hypertens 2001; **15**:669–76.

Design

Randomized.

Sample size (n)

1205 (prevalence study) and 106 (intervention study).

Questions addressed

- To compare the effects of balloon angioplasty and antihypertensive medication on BP in patients with ≥50% atherosclerotic RAS.
- To study the usefulness of standardized 2-drug regimens for identifying drug-resistant hypertension as a predictor of RAS.

1° endpoint

BP.

Results

- Prevalence study: 772 patients were included in the randomization. Drug-resistant hypertension was observed in 32.2% of patients receiving amlodipine with/without atenolol and in 41.7% of those receiving enalapril with/without hydrochlorothiazide ($p = 0.006$). However, there was no significant difference between the groups in the incidence of RAS.
- Intervention study: at 3 and 12 months, BP was similar in the 2 groups as was drug dose and kidney function. 22 patients in the medical treatment group underwent angioplasty because of persistent hypertension.

Dublin Outcome Study

Trial name
Dublin Outcome Study.

Reference
Hypertens 2005; **46**:156–61.

Design
Prospective.

Sample size (n)
5292.

Question addressed
The additional predictive value of ABPM over clinic BP in predicting outcome.

1° endpoint
Prediction of mortality.

Results
Ambulatory measurements are superior to clinic measurements in predicting CV mortality and night-time BP is a better predictor than daytime pressure.

ELITE

Trial name

Evaluation of Losartan In The Elderly.

Reference

Lancet 1997; **349**:747–52.

Design

Randomized, double-blind, controlled, parallel-group.

Sample size (n)

722 patients.

Question addressed

To determine whether specific angiotensin II receptor blockade with losartan offers safety and efficacy advantages in the treatment of heart failure over ACE inhibition with captopril in the elderly.

1° endpoint

Mortality and morbidity.

Results

Death and/or hospital admission for heart failure occurred in 9.4% of the losartan and 13.2% of the captopril patients (RR 32%; 95% CI –4% to +55%; p = 0.075). This RR was primarily the result of a ↓ in all-cause mortality (4.8% vs. 8.7%; RR 46%; 95% CI 5–69%; p = 0.035). Admissions with heart failure were the same in both groups as was improvement in NYHA class from baseline. Admission to hospital for any reason was less frequent with losartan treatment.

EPHESUS

Trial name
Eplerenone Post-AMI Heart failure Efficacy and Survival Study.

Reference
Cardiovasc Drugs Ther 2001; **15**:79–87.

Design
Randomized, double-blind, placebo-controlled.

Sample size (n)
6632.

Question addressed
To compare the effect of eplerenone plus standard therapy to placebo plus standard therapy on mortality and morbidity in patients with heart failure after AMI.

1° endpoint
Mortality and morbidity.

Results
All-cause mortality was lower in patients on eplerenone placebo (14.4 vs. 16.7%, $p = 0.008$). The combined incidence of CV mortality or hospitalization for CV events was also lower in the active group (26.7% vs. 30.0%, $p = 0.002$).

EWPHE

Trial name

European Working Party on High Blood Pressure in the Elderly.

Reference

Lancet 1985; **1**:1349–54.

Design

Randomized, double blind, placebo-controlled.

Sample size (n)

840.

Question addressed

To compare the effect of hydrochlorothiazide and triamterene treatment versus placebo on mortality in the elderly.

1° endpoint

Mortality and morbidity.

Results

There was a 21/10 difference in BP between active and placebo arms. CV mortality was reduced in the actively treated group (–38%, $p = 0.023$), owing to a reduction in cardiac deaths (–47%, $p = 0.048$) and a non-significant ↓ in cerebrovascular mortality (–43%, $p = 0.15$). In the patients randomized to active treatment there were 29 fewer CV events and 14 fewer CV deaths per 1000 patient years during the double-blind part of the trial.

EUROASPIRE II

Trial name

European Action on Secondary Prevention through Intervention to Reduce Events II.

Reference

Eur Heart J 2001; **22**:554–72.

Design

Observational.

Sample size (n)

8181.

Question addressed

To determine in patients with established CHD whether the Joint European Societies' recommendations on coronary prevention are being followed in clinical practice.

1° endpoint

Practice audit across Europe of CV risk factors.

Results

- 5556 patients; 21% smoked, 31% were obese, 50% had SBP ≥140mmHg and/or DBP ≥90mmHg, 58% had serum total cholesterol ≥ 5mmol/L, and 20% reported diabetes mellitus. 87% of diabetic patients had plasma glucose >6.0mmol/L.
- There was variable use of proven therapies—most were on aspirin/other antiplatelets and β-blockers but a smaller proportion on ACEIS and statins (data are for admission, at discharge and at interview):
    - Aspirin/other antiplatelets: 47%, 90% and 86%.
    - β-blockers 44%, 66%, and 63%.
    - ACEI 24%, 38%, and 38%.
    - Lipid lowering 26%, 43%, and 61%.
- The proportion of patients overall taking statins was 55.3%.

HOPE

Trial name
Heart Outcomes Prevention Evaluation study.

Reference
NEJM 2000; **342**:145–53.

Design
Randomized, double-blind, placebo-controlled parallel-group, 2 × 2 factorial.

Sample size (n)
9541.

Question addressed
Does ramipril reduce the incidence of MI, stroke or CV death?

1° endpoint
Mortality and morbidity.

Results
- There was a significant reduction in events in the ramipril group for the 1° endpoint (14.0% vs. 17.8% placebo, p <0.001).
- Active therapy reduced MI (9.9% vs. 12.3%), stroke (3.4% vs. 4.9%) and CV death (6.1% vs. 8.1%), compared to placebo (p <0.001 for all endpoints).

HOT

Trial name

Hypertension Optimal Treatment Study.

Reference

Lancet 1998; **351**:1755–62.

Design

Randomized, open, single-blind (antihypertensive treatment) and double-blind (aspirin).

Sample size (n)

18,790.

Question addressed

- Does target DBP affect major CV events (non-fatal, acute, and silent MI, non-fatal stroke, and all CV causes of death)?
- 2°: does low-dose aspirin, in addition to antihypertensive therapy reduce the incidence of major CV events?

1° endpoint

Mortality and morbidity

Results

- The DBP was reduced to 85.2, 83.2, and 81.1mmHg in the target groups ≤90, ≤85 and ≤80mmHg, respectively.
- The lowest incidence of major CV events occurred at a mean achieved DBP of 82.6mmHg and SBP of 138.5mmHg and the lowest risk of CV mortality at DBP 86.5mmHg and at SBP 138.8mmHg.
- There was no J-shaped relationship with mortality.
- There was a 51% reduction in major CV events in diabetics with a target ≤80mmHg compared to ≤90mmHg.
- Aspirin reduced major CV events by 15% and all MI by 36%.
- There was no effect on the incidence of stroke or fatal bleeds by aspirin, but non-fatal major bleeds were twice as common with aspirin

HYVET

Trial name
Hypertension in the Very Elderly Trial.

Reference
NEJM 2008; **358**:1887–98.

Design
Randomized, double-blind, placebo-controlled.

Sample size (n)
3845.

Question addressed
To determine whether active treatment (with indapamide ± perindopril) of hypertension in patients >80 years with SBP >160mmHg to target 150/80 reduces stroke.

1° endpoint
Mortality and morbidity.

Results
- 30% reduction in the rate of fatal or non-fatal stroke (p=0.06), 39% reduction in the rate of death from stroke (p=0.05), 21% reduction in death from any cause (p=0.02), 23% reduction in the CV death (p=0.06), and 64% reduction in the rate of heart failure (p<0.001).
- Careful BP lowering in the very elderly is beneficial.

IDNT

Trial name
Irbesartan type 2 Diabetic Nephropathy Trial.

Reference
NEJM 2001; **345**:851–60.

Design
Randomized, double-blind, placebo-controlled.

Sample size (n)
1715.

Question addressed
To determine whether irbesartan and amlodipine slow the progression of nephropathy in patients with type 2 diabetes independent of their ability to lower SBP.

1° endpoint
Mortality and morbidity.

Results
- Irbesartan reduced doubling of serum creatinine, end-stage renal failure and death from any cause by 20% compared to placebo (p = 0.02) and 23% lower than in the amlodipine group (p = 0.006). These differences were not explained by changes in BP.
- The serum creatinine concentration ↑ 24% more slowly in the irbesartan group than in the placebo group (p = 0.008) and 21% more slowly than in the amlodipine group (p = 0.02).

INTERSALT

Trial name
Intersalt: an international study of electrolyte excretion and blood pressure.

Reference
BMJ 1988; **297**:319–28.
Hypertension 1991; 17(1 Suppl.):I9–15.

Design
Observational.

Sample size (n)
10,079.

Question addressed
Relationship between electrolyte excretion and BP.

1° endpoint
Correlation between sodium excretion and BP.

Results
- Na^+ excretion ranged from 0.2 to 242mmol/24h. In individual subjects (within centres) it was significantly related to BP. In 48 centres of 52, Na^+ was significantly related to the slope of BP with age but not to median BP or prevalence of high BP.
- K^+ excretion was negatively correlated with BP in individual subjects after adjustment for confounding variables. BMI and heavy alcohol intake had strong, significant independent relations with BP in individual subjects.

INSIGHT

Trial name

International Nifedipine GITS Study Intervention as a Goal in Hypertension Treatment.

Reference

Lancet 2000; **356**:366–72.

Design

Randomized, double-blind, parallel-group.

Sample size (n)

6321.

Question addressed

To compare 1° endpoint in high-risk hypertensive patients treated with nifedipine GITS or amiloride plus hydrochlorothiazide.

1° endpoint

Mortality and morbidity.

Results

- Mean BP fell by 35/17mmHg. The combined incidence of MI, heart failure, stroke, and CV death was not different for nifedipine GITS or co-amilozide ($p = 0.34$).
- Total mortality was the same in both groups (4.8%) but there were fewer vascular deaths than non-vascular deaths

ISIS IV

Trial name

ISIS-4: a randomized factorial trial assessing early oral captopril, oral mononitrate, and intravenous magnesium sulphate in 58,050 patients with suspected acute MI. ISIS-4 (Fourth International Study of Infarct Survival) Collaborative Group.

Reference

Lancet 1995; **345**:669–85.

Design

Randomized, 2 × 2 × 2 factorial, placebo controlled.

Sample size (n)

58,050.

Question addressed

To determine if an ACEI (captopril), nitrate, or magnesium alters mortality in patients post MI.

1° endpoint

Mortality and morbidity.

Results

ACEI: small but significant reduction in 5-week mortality with survival advantage maintained at 1 year especially in high-risk patients. Neither nitrates nor magnesium caused significant changes to the endpoints.

LIFE

Trial name

Losartan Intervention For Endpoint reduction in hypertension.

Reference

Lancet 2002; **359**:995–1003.

Design

Randomized, double-blind, double-dummy, parallel-group.

Sample size (n)

9193.

Question addressed

Effects of losartan vs. atenolol on CV mortality and morbidity in hypertensive patients with LVH.

1° endpoint

Mortality and morbidity.

Results

- There was no significant difference in brachial BP reduction between the 2 groups.
- Losartan had a lower 1° endpoint than atenolol ($p = 0.021$).
- New-onset diabetes mellitus was 25% lower with losartan and there was greater reduction of LVH ($p < 0.0001$).

MAGPIE

Trial name
Magnesium sulphate for prevention of eclampsia.

Reference
Lancet 2002; **359**:1877–90.

Design
Randomized, double-blind, placebo-controlled.

Sample size (n)
10,110.

Question addressed
Does magnesium sulphate reduce the risk of eclampsia?

1° endpoint
Mortality and morbidity

Results
- Active treatment reduced the risk of eclampsia ($p<0.0001$) and maternal mortality.
- There was no difference in neonatal mortality or any antihypertensive effects.

MRC Elderly

Trial name

Medical Research Council trial of treatment of hypertension in older adults.

Reference

BMJ 1992; **304**:405–12
Clin Exp Hypertens 1993; **15**:941–2.

Design

Randomized, single-blind, placebo-controlled, parallel-group.

Sample size (n)

4396.

Questions addressed

- Do antihypertensives in patients (65–74 years) reduce mortality and morbidity due to stroke and CHD and mortality from all causes?
- 2° endpoint: to compare the effects of hydrochlorothiazide (or amiloride) and atenolol and to see whether responses to treatment differed between men and women.

1° endpoint

Mortality and morbidity.

Results

- Active treatment reduced BP more than placebo.
- Patients in the active treatment groups had a 25% reduction in stroke, a 19% reduction in coronary events, and a 17% reduction in all CV events.
- The diuretic group had significantly reduced risks of stroke, coronary events, and all CV events compared to the placebo group.
- The beta-blocker group showed no significant reduction in these endpoints.

MRC/BHF HPS

Trial name

Medical Research Council and British Heart Foundation Heart Protection Study.

Reference

Lancet 2002; **360**:7–22.

Design

Randomized, placebo-controlled, 2 × 2 factorial.

Sample size (n)

20,536.

Question addressed

To assess the effects on mortality and major morbidity of cholesterol-lowering therapy and of antioxidant vitamin supplementation in patients at high risk of CVD.

1° endpoint

Mortality and morbidity.

Results

- There were fewer deaths in the simvastatin group compared to placebo (1328 [12.9%] vs. 1507 [14.7%], p = 0.0003); the death rate from vascular causes was also significantly reduced (7.6% vs. 9.1% in the placebo group, p <0.0001).
- Coronary death rate was 5.7% and 6.9%, respectively (p = 0.0005), and the death rate from other vascular causes was 1.9% and 2.2%, respectively (p = 0.07).
- First non-fatal MI rate (3.5% vs. 5.6%, p <0.0001) and first stroke rate (4.3% vs. 5.7%, p <0.0001) were also markedly reduced as were the need for revascularization (9.1% vs. 11.7%; p <0.0001).
- Vitamin supplementation did not alter all-cause mortality (14.1% vs. 13.5%), deaths due to vascular (8.6% vs. 8.2%) or non-vascular (5.5% vs. 5.3%) causes, nor the incidences of non-fatal MI, coronary death, non-fatal/fatal stroke, revascularization procedure, or cancer incidence.

MRFIT

Trial name
Multiple Risk Factor Intervention Trial.

Reference
JAMA 1982; **248**:1465–77.

Design
Randomized, open, usual care controlled.

Sample size (n)
12,866.

Question addressed
To test the efficacy of a multifactor intervention programme in CHD.

1° endpoint
Mortality.

Results
- Mortality from CHD was 17.9 deaths/1000 in the special intervention group and 19.3 deaths/1000 in the group receiving usual care.
- Total mortality rates were 41.2 deaths/1000 in the special intervention group and 40.4 deaths/1000 in the group receiving usual care.
- At 10.5 years, CHD mortality was still 10.6% lower in the special intervention group compared to the usual care group, and the AMI rate was 24.3% lower.
- At 16 years, the differences remained about the same. Only the differences in AMI rate were statistically significant.

NHANES III

Trial name

National Health and Nutrition Examination Survey III.

Reference

Hypertens 2001; **37**:869–74.

Design

Observational.

Sample size (n)

19,661.

Questions addressed

- To assess frequency of ISH and other subtypes of hypertension, hypertension awareness, and treatment target goals.
- Does subtypes and staging vary between age groups?

1° endpoint

Prevalence.

Results

ISH commonest in older groups (aged 50–59, frequency 87%). This requires greater attention to treatment of SBP.

NORDIL

Trial name
Nordic Diltiazem study.

Reference
Lancet 2000; **356**:359–65.

Design
Randomized, open, blinded-endpoint, parallel-group.

Sample size (n)
10,881.

Question addressed
Effects of diltiazem on CV morbidity and mortality compared to other antihypertensive agents.

1° endpoint
Mortality and morbidity.

Results
- SBP and DBP were lowered in the diltiazem and β-blocker/diuretic groups (reduction, 20.3/18.7 vs. 23.3/18.7mmHg; $p < 0.001$ for SBP reduction)
- There was no significant difference between the groups for the 1° endpoint of fatal and non-fatal MI but there was a difference in favour of diltiazem for fatal and non-fatal stroke ($p = 0.04$).
- Diltiazem was as effective as other therapies in the combined 1° endpoint of fatal/non-fatal MI and stroke or other CV death.

ONTARGET

Trial name

Ongoing Telmisartan Alone and in Combination with Ramipril Global Endpoint Trial.

Reference

NEJM 2008; **358**:1547–59.

Design

Double blind, randomized

Sample size (n)

25,620

Question addressed

Effects of ACE and ARA or the combination in patients who have vascular disease or high-risk diabetes without heart failure on mortality and morbidity. The 1° composite outcome was death from CV causes, MI, stroke, or hospitalization for heart failure.

1° endpoint

Mortality and morbidity.

Results

- Mean BP was lower in both the telmisartan group (a 0.9/0.6mmHg greater reduction) and the combination-therapy group (a 2.4/1.4mmHg greater reduction) than in the ramipril group.
- Telmisartan caused lower rates of cough (1.1% vs. 4.2%, p <0.001) and angioedema (0.1% vs. 0.3%, p = 0.01) and a higher rate of hypotensive symptoms (2.6% vs. 1.7%, p <0.001); the rate of syncope was the same.
- In the combination-therapy group, the 1° outcome occurred in 1386 patients (16.3%; RR, 0.99; 95% CI, 0.92–1.07); as compared with the ramipril group, there was an ↑ risk of hypotensive symptoms (4.8% vs. 1.7%, p <0.001), syncope (0.3% vs. 0.2%, p = 0.03), and renal dysfunction (13.5% vs. 10.2%, p <0.001).
- Telmisartan was equivalent to ramipril in patients with vascular disease or high-risk diabetes and was associated with less angioedema.
- The combination of the 2 drugs was associated with more adverse events without an ↑ in benefit.

PATS

Trial name

Post-stroke antihypertensive treatment study.

Reference

Chin Med J 1995; **108**:710–7.

Design

Randomized, double-blind, placebo-controlled.

Sample size (n)

5665.

Question addressed

Does antihypertensive therapy with a diuretic after a stroke reduce subsequent events?

1° endpoint

Mortality and morbidity.

Results

BP reduction by 5/2mmHg with indapamide in patients with a history of stroke/TIA reduced the incidence of fatal/non-fatal stroke by 29%.

PROGRESS

Trial name
Perindopril Protection against Recurrent Stroke Study.

Reference
Lancet 2001; **358**:1033–41.

Design
Randomized, double-blind, placebo-controlled.

Sample size (n)
6105.

Question addressed
To determine the effects of BP reduction on stroke risk in patients with a history of cerebrovascular disease.

1° endpoint
Mortality and morbidity.

Results
- Treatment reduced BP by 9/4mmHg compared to placebo.
- 10% of patients on active treatment suffered a stroke compared to 14% on placebo (RR reduction 28%; p <0.0001).
- The risk of total major vascular events in the active treatment group was 15% compared to 20% in the placebo group.
- Active treatment also reduced the risk of stroke in hypertensive and non-hypertensive subgroups (p <0.01).
- Perindopril plus indapamide reduced SBP by 12mmHg and DBP by 5mmHg, and the risk of stroke by 43%.
- Perindopril alone reduced SBP by 5mmHg and DBP by 3mmHg, *but not the risk of stroke.*

PRAISE

Trial name
Prospective Randomized Amlodipine Survival Evaluation.

Reference
NEJM 1996; **335**:1107–14.

Design
Randomized, double-blind, placebo-controlled, parallel-group.

Sample size (n)
1153.

Question addressed
To assess the efficacy and safety of amlodipine in patients with severe chronic heart failure.

1° endpoint
Mortality and morbidity.

Results
- A 1° fatal or non-fatal event occurred in 42% of patients in the placebo group and 39% in the amlodipine group.
- The mortality rate was 38% in the placebo group and 33% in the amlodipine group.
- However, there was no difference in these rates between the amlodipine and placebo treatments in patients with ischaemic conditions; the risk of death and the combined risk of fatal and non-fatal events were reduced only in patients with non-ischaemic dilated cardiomyopathy.
- Oedema and orthostatic hypotension were more frequent in the amlodipine group.

RALES

Trial name
Randomized Aldactone Evaluation Study.

Reference
NEJM 1999; **341**:709–17.

Design
Randomized, double-blind, placebo-controlled.

Sample size (n)
1663.

Question addressed
To test the hypothesis that treatment with spironolactone would reduce all-cause mortality in patients with severe heart failure who were receiving standard therapy.

1° endpoint
Mortality.

Results
Spironolactone had a significantly reduced all-cause mortality rate compared to placebo (35% vs. 46%, RR 0.70, p <0.001).

REIN

Trial name

Ramipril Efficacy In Nephropathy.

Reference

J Nephrol 1991; **3**:193–202.

Design

Randomized, double-blind, placebo-controlled (2 years) plus open (3-year extension).

Sample size (n)

352.

Question addressed

- Effects of ramipril vs. placebo on the rate of decline of GFR in patients with chronic non-diabetic nephropathy and proteinuria.
- 2° endpoints: 24-h proteinuria, end-stage renal events plus CV events and death, and lipid profile.

1° endpoint

Morbidity.

Results

- Mean rate of GFR decline was significantly lower in the ramipril-treated patients than in the placebo group, 0.53 vs. 0.88mL/min/month (p = 0.03).
- Urinary protein excretion ↓ significantly (p <0.01) by month 1 in the ramipril group and remained lower than baseline throughout the study period (no change in placebo group).
- The need for transplantation or dialysis and doubling of serum creatinine were significantly ↓ in the ramipril group (p = 0.02).
- BP control and the overall number of CV events were similar in the 2 treatment groups.
- Baseline urinary protein excretion rate was the best single predictor of renal disease progression.
- Progression to end-stage renal failure (RR 2.72; p = 0.01) and progression to overt proteinuria (RR 2.40; p = 0.005) were significantly more common in the placebo group than in the ramipril group.
- Ramipril significantly ↓ proteinuria by 13% whilst placebo ↑ it by 15% (p = 0.003). The rate of decline of GFR (p = 0.0001) and the incidence of end-stage renal failure (RR 5.44; p = 0.0001) were much higher in stratum 2 than in stratum 1.

RENAAL

Trial name

Effects of Losartan on renal and CV outcomes in patients with Type 2 Diabetes and nehropathy.

Reference

NEJM 2001; **345**:861–9.

Design

Randomized, double blind.

Sample size (n)

1513.

Question addressed

The role of the angiotensin-II–receptor antagonist losartan in patients with type 2 diabetes and nephropathy. 1° outcome was the composite of a doubling of the base-line serum creatinine concentration, end-stage renal disease, or death.
2°end points included a composite of morbidity and mortality from CV causes, proteinuria and the rate of progression of renal disease.

1° endpoint

Morbidity.

Results

- Losartan reduced the incidence of a doubling of the serum creatinine concentration (RR 25%; p = 0.006) and ESRD (RR 28%; p=0.002) but had no effect on the rate of death. This benefit was independent of changes in BP.
- The rate of 1st hospitalization for heart failure was significantly lower with losartan (RR 32%; p=0.005).
- The level of proteinuria declined by 35% with losartan (p <0.001 for the comparison with placebo).
- Losartan conferred significant renal benefits in patients with type 2 diabetes and nephropathy and it was generally well tolerated.

SENIORS

Trial name

The effect of nebivolol on mortality and CV hospital admission in elderly patients with heart failure.

Reference

Eur Heart J 2005; **26**: 215–25.

Design

Randomized, double blind, placebo controlled, parallel group.

Sample size (n)

2128.

Question addressed

Effects of nebivolol on elderly heart failure patients.

1° endpoint

Mortality or CV hospitalization.

Results

Nebivolol significantly reduced all cause mortality or CV hospitalization (31% vs. 35%, $p = 0.039$).

SHARP

Trial name
Stop Hypertension with the Acupuncture Research Program (SHARP): results of a randomized, controlled clinical trial.

Reference
Hypertension 2006; **48**:838–45.

Design
Prospective, double bline, randomized, sham controlled, parallel group.

Sample size (n)
192.

Question addressed
To determine if acupuncture can effectively treat hypertension.

1° endpoint
BP.

Results
- The mean BP ↓ from baseline to 10 weeks, the 1° end point, did not differ significantly between participants randomly assigned to active (individualized and standardized) versus sham acupuncture (SBP: –3.56 versus –3.84mmHg, respectively; 95% CI for the difference: –4.0 to 4.6mmHg; p = 0.90; DBP: –4.32 versus –2.81mmHg, 95% CI for the difference: –3.6 to 0.6mmHg; p = 0.16).
- Categorizing participants by age, race, gender, baseline BP, history of antihypertensive use, obesity, or 1° traditional Chinese medicine diagnosis did not reveal any subgroups for which the benefits of active acupuncture differed significantly from sham acupuncture.
- Active acupuncture provided no greater benefit than invasive sham acupuncture in reducing SBP or DBP.

SHEP

Trial name
Systolic Hypertension in the Elderly Program.

Reference
JAMA 1991; **265**:3255–64.

Design
Randomized, double-blind, placebo-controlled.

Sample size (n)
4736.

Question addressed
Does antihypertensive drug treatment with chlortalidone reduce the risk of total stroke (both non-fatal and fatal) with ISH, aged ≥ 60 years?

1° endpoint
Mortality and morbidity.

Results
- At 5 years, there was a 12/4mmHg difference in BP between the groups (lower in the active group).
- The 5-year incidence of total stroke was 5.2% in the active treatment group and 8.2% in the placebo group (RR 0.64, p = 0.0003).
- The RR of clinical non-fatal MI plus coronary death, which was the 2° endpoint, was 0.73. Major CV events were also reduced (RR 0.68). The RR of death from all causes was 0.87.
- Patients >75 years and women underwent fewer intensive CV interventions than did patients 60–75 years and men.
- Active treatment was significantly associated with ↓ use of coronary artery by pass graft and percutaneous transluminal coronary angioplastyin patients <75 years with CHD.
- The incidence of both haemorrhagic (9 vs. 19; risk ratio = 0.46) and ischaemic (85 vs. 132; risk ratio = 0.63) strokes were reduced in the active treatment group.
- The effect of treatment on haemorrhagic strokes was seen in the 1st year, but the effect on ischaemic strokes was not seen until the 2nd year.

SOLVD

Trial name

Studies Of Left Ventricular Dysfunction.

Reference

NEJM 1991; **325**: 293–302.

Design

Randomized, double-blind, placebo-controlled.

Sample size (n)

4228.

Questions addressed

- Does enalapril improve long-term survival in patients with left ventricular dysfunction with and without a history of overt congestive heart failure?
- 2° objective: to demonstrate its effects in different subgroups of patients, e.g. group according to plasma sodium, vasodilator treatment, ejection fraction, aetiology, and NYHA class. Also to study effects on left ventricular function and volume, arrhythmias, quality of life, and pharmacoeconomy.

1° endpoint

Mortality.

Results

- Prevention trial: the reduction in mortality from CV causes was larger but still not statistically significant. However, the combined incidence of death and development of overt congestive heart failure showed a risk reduction of 29% ($p < 0.001$).
- Treatment trial: there were 510 deaths in the placebo group and 452 in the enalapril group. This represents a risk reduction of 16% ($p = 0.0036$). The greatest reduction was seen in the number of deaths attributed to progressive heart failure.
- The following analyses were performed in patients from both trials:
  - No apparent changes in quality of life for ≥1 year and only modest benefits in quality of life occurred in the enalapril-treated patients in the treatment trial
  - No significant differences in ventricular arrhythmia development over 1 year.
  - Left ventricular end-diastolic and end-systolic volumes ↑ in placebo- but not active treatment ($p < 0.05$ for both). Left ventricular mass tended to ↑ in placebo patients and to ↓ in enalapril-treated patients ($p \leq 0.001$)

- For the 48 months within the treatment trial, study participants who received enalapril lived an average of 0.16 undiscounted years longer. The lifetime projection of this indicated that participants who received enalapril would be expected to live, on average, 0.40 years longer than those on placebo. Within the trial, the patient receiving enalapril costed on the average about US$720 less than the patient receiving placebo, due to higher costs for hospitalizations. In lifetime projections, the costs per year of life saved and per quality-adjusted year of life saved were estimated to be US$80 and US$115, respectively.

STOP HYPERTENSION 2

Trial name
Swedish Trial in Old Patients with Hypertension 2.

Reference
Lancet 1999; **354**:1751–6.

Design
Randomized, open, blinded endpoint (PROBE design).

Sample size (n)
6614.

Question addressed
To evaluate classical antihypertensive agents, diuretics, and β-blockers, vs. the newer antihypertensive agents, lisinopril, enalapril, isradipine, and felodipine, on CV mortality and events in elderly hypertensives.

1° endpoint
Mortality and morbidity.

Results
- There were no significant differences between the groups in fatal CV events (β-blocker/diuretic group vs. calcium antagonist and ACEI group, RR 0.99; $p = 0.89$).
- The combined endpoint of fatal and non-fatal stroke, fatal and non-fatal MI, and other CV mortality was also not significant comparing conventional therapy vs. newer agents (RR 0.96; $p = 0.49$).

Syst-China

Trial name

Systolic hypertension in China.

Reference

J Hum Hypertens 1998; **16**:1823–9.

Design

Randomized, double-blind, placebo-controlled.

Sample size (n)

2394.

Questions addressed

- To assess whether nitrendipine, if necessary combined with captopril and hydrochlorothiazide, is suitable for maintaining long-term BP control in older Chinese patients with ISH.
- Furthermore, whether this therapy can reduce the incidence of stroke and other CV complications.

1° endpoint

Mortality and morbidity.

Results

- Therapy reduced BP by 9/3mmHg more in than the placebo group.
- This translated to a significant reduction in stroke by 38% ($p = 0.01$), stroke mortality by 58% ($p = 0.02$), all-cause mortality by 39% ($p = 0.003$), CV mortality by 39% ($p = 0.03$), and all fatal and non-fatal CV endpoints by 37% ($p = 0.004$).

Syst-Eur

Trial name

Systolic hypertension in Europe.

Reference

Lancet 1997; **350**:757–64.

Design

Randomized, double-blind, placebo-controlled.

Sample size (n)

4695.

Question addressed

Does antihypertensive treatment (nitrendipine) in elderly patients with ISH reduce CV events, primarily fatal and non-fatal stroke?

1° endpoint

Mortality and morbidity.

Results

- Treatment reduced all strokes by 42% (p = 0.003) and non-fatal strokes by 44% (p = 0.007). However, there was no effect on the incidence of TIA by active treatment (–12%; p = 0.62).
- In the active treatment group, all fatal and non-fatal cardiac endpoints, including sudden death, ↓ by 26% (p = 0.03).

THOP

Trial name
Treatment of Hypertension according to home or Office blood Pressure.

Reference
Am J Hypertens 2003; **16**:63A.

Design
Randomized, parallel-group.

Sample size (n)
400.

Question addressed
Is antihypertensive treatment guided by self-measured BP more beneficial than treatment based on clinic BP?

1° endpoint
Morbidity.

Results
- BP was higher in patients with home measurement than in patients with office measurement ($p<0.001$).
- Antihypertensive treatment was discontinued significantly more frequently in patients with home measurement than in patients with office measurement (25.2% vs. 12.3%; $p = 0.001$).
- Fewer patients with home measurement progressed to multiple drug treatment than patients with office measurement (38.7% vs. 46.4%; $p = 0.08$).

TNT

Trial name

Treating to New Targets.

Reference

NEJM 2005; **352**:1425–35.

Design

Randomized, double blind, parallel-group.

Sample size (n)

10,001.

Question addressed

To assess efficacy and safety of moderate and intensive statin therapy with a goal of reducing CV risk by reducing LDL cholesterol below recommended targets of 2.6mmol/L in patients with CHD.

1° endpoint

Mortality and morbidity.

Results

- Mean cholesterol levels were 2.6mmol/L with atorvastatin 10mg/day and 2.0mmol/L with atorvastatin 80 mg/day.
- 1° endpoint of CV death, non-fatal MI, resuscitation after cardiac arrest, fatal or non-fatal stroke occurred less in the 80mg/day group (10.9% vs. 8.7%, RRR 22%, $p < 0.001$).
- There was no significant difference in overall mortality between the 2 groups.

TONE

Trial name

Sodium Reduction and Weight Loss in the Treatment of Hypertension in Older Persons. A Randomized Controlled Trial of Nonpharmacologic Interventions in the Elderly (TONE).

Reference

JAMA 1998; **279**:839–46.

Design

Randomized.

Sample size (n)

875.

Question addressed

To determine whether weight loss or reduced sodium intake is effective in the treatment of older persons with hypertension.

1° endpoint

Morbidity.

Results

- The combined outcome measure was less frequent among those assigned vs. not assigned to reduced sodium intake (relative HR, 0.69; 95% CI, 0.59–0.81; p <.001) and, in obese participants, among those assigned vs. not assigned to weight loss (relative HR, 0.70; 95% CI, 0.57–0.87; p <.001).
- Relative to usual care, HRs among the obese participants were 0.60 (95% CI, 0.45–0.80; p <.001) for reduced sodium intake alone, 0.64 (95% CI, 0.49–0.85; p = 0.002) for weight loss alone, and 0.47 (95% CI, 0.35–0.64; p <0.001) for reduced sodium intake and weight loss combined.
- The frequency of CV events during follow-up was similar in each of the 6 treatment groups.
- Reduced sodium intake and weight loss constitute a feasible, effective, and safe non-pharmacologic therapy of hypertension in older persons.

UKPDS/HDS

Trial name

UK Prospective Diabetes Study – Hypertension in Diabetes Study.

Referece

BMJ 1998; **317**:713–20.

Design

Randomized, open, factorial.

Sample size (n)

- 4209 in UKPDS.
- 1148 in HDS.

Questions addressed

To determine whether improved blood glucose control and tight control of BP will prevent complications and reduce morbidity and mortality in patients with type 2 diabetes, and to determine which, if any, therapies have a particular advantage in improving prognosis.

Results

- Over 10 years, intensive blood glucose control significantly reduced HbA1c compared to conventional treatment (7.0% vs. 7.9%; $p < 0.0001$), with non-significant reductions in the risk of diabetes-related death (10%) and all-cause mortality (6%), and a reduction in risk of MI of borderline significance ($p = 0.052$).
- None of the intensive antidiabetic agents showed an advantage over the others.
- Mortality in overweight patients receiving metformin was 36% lower than in overweight patients receiving conventional treatment ($p = 0.011$), with a significant 39% reduction in the incidence of MI ($p = 0.01$).
- Tight control of BP significantly reduced the risk of diabetes-related death by 32% ($p = 0.019$), of any diabetes-related endpoint by 24% ($p = 0.0046$), and of stroke by 44% ($p = 0.013$).
- The risk of MI was reduced in the tight BP control group by 21%, and the combined risk of all macrovascular diseases (including MI, sudden death, stroke, and peripheral vascular disease) was significantly reduced by 34% ($p = 0.019$).
- The risk of heart failure was significantly reduced by 56% ($p = 0.0043$) by tight BP control.
- By 7.5 years, the tight BP control group showed a 48% reduction in risk of a Q-wave ECG abnormality ($p = 0.007$).
- BP reduction is key to reducing the risk of either single or aggregate macrovascular endpoints.

VA Cooperative Study

Trial name
Veteran's Administration Co-operative Study.

Reference
JAMA 1967; **202**:1028–34.

Design
Randomized, double blind, placebo controlled.

Sample size (n)
143.

Question addressed
Does antihypertensive treatment (hydrochlorothiazide, reserpine, and hydralazine) reduce events in patients with hypertension with end-organ damage (DBP 115–129mmHg).

1° endpoint
Mortality.

Results
There were 27 deaths in the placebo arm and only 2 in the active arm ($p < 0.01$).

VALHEFT

Trial name
Valsartan Heart Failure Trial.

Reference
NEJM 2001; **345**:1667–75.

Design
Randomized, placebo-controlled.

Sample size (n)
5010.

Question addressed
To investigate the effects of valsartan on mortality, morbidity, and quality of life in patients with chronic heart failure treated with ACEIs with or without background β-blocker therapy.

1° endpoint
Mortality and morbidity.

Results
- The rate of all-cause mortality was similar in the two groups.
- Valsartan significantly reduced combined mortality and morbidity from heart failure ($p = 0.009$).
- Valsartan also improved NYHA class, ejection fraction, signs and symptoms of heart failure, and quality of life compared to placebo ($p < 0.01$).
- A post-hoc analysis of the data in subgroups defined according to baseline treatment with ACEIs or β-blockers showed that valsartan had a favourable effect in patients who received none or one of these drugs, but had an adverse effect on mortality in patients who received both types of drugs.

VALUE

Trial name
Valsartan Antihypertensive Long-term Use Evaluation.

Reference
Lancet 2004; **363**:2022–31.

Design
Randomized, double-blind, parallel-group.

Sample size (n)
15,245.

Question addressed
Is valsartan more effective than amlodipine in reducing cardiac mortality and morbidity for the same level of BP control?

1° endpoint
Mortality and morbidity.

Results
There were no differences between the treatment groups in either cardiac mortality ($p = 0.90$) or cardiac morbidity ($p = 0.71$).

Index